HEALTHY INSPIRATION

absolute PILATES

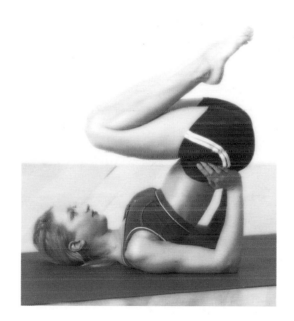

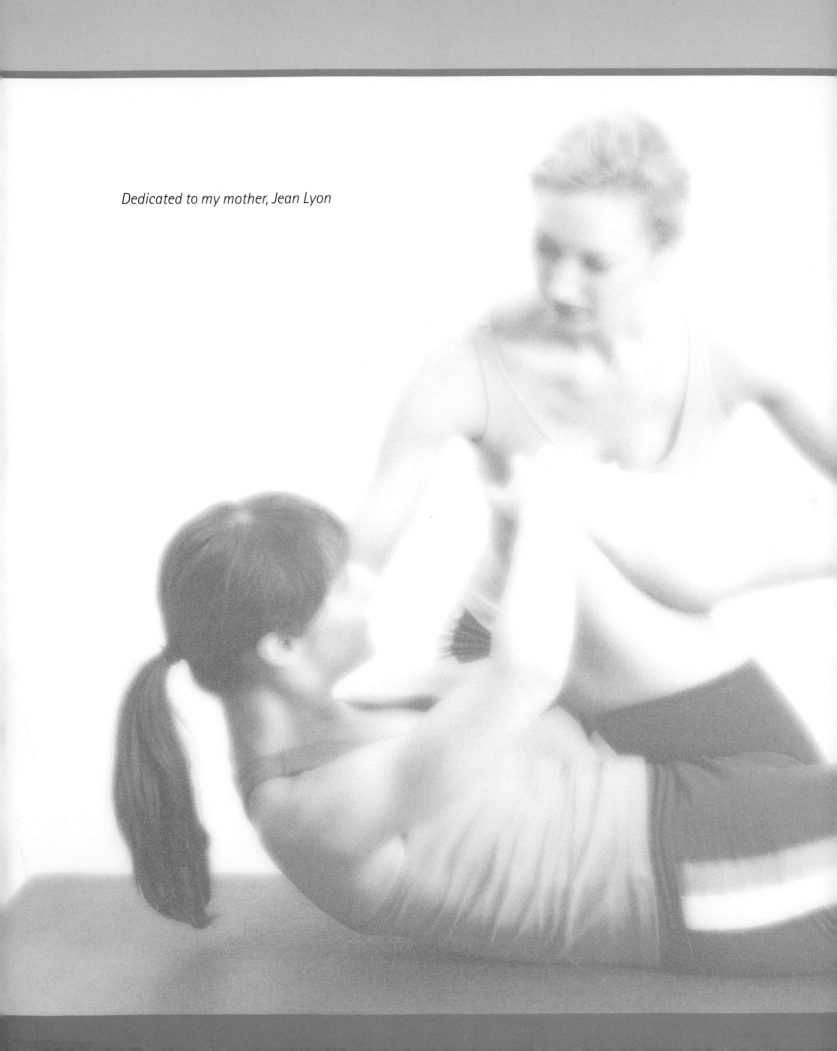

Dedicated to my mother, Jean Lyon

HEALTHY INSPIRATION

absolute PILATES

Caron Bosler

Published by SILVERDALE BOOKS
An imprint of Bookmart Ltd
Registered number 2372865
Trading as Bookmart Ltd
Blaby Road
Wigston
Leicester LE18 4SE

© 2005 D&S Books Ltd

D&S Books Ltd
Kerswell,
Parkham Ash, Bideford
Devon, England
EX39 5PR

e-mail us at:- enquiries@d-sbooks.co.uk

This edition printed 2005

ISBN 1-84509-272-4

DS0116. Healthy inspirations - Pilates

Creative Director: Sarah King
Editor: Nicky Barber
Project editor: Judith Millidge
Designer: Debbie Fisher
Photographer: Paul Forrester

Fonts: Rotis Sans Serif and Vag Rounded

Printed in China

1 3 5 7 9 10 8 6 4 2

Contents

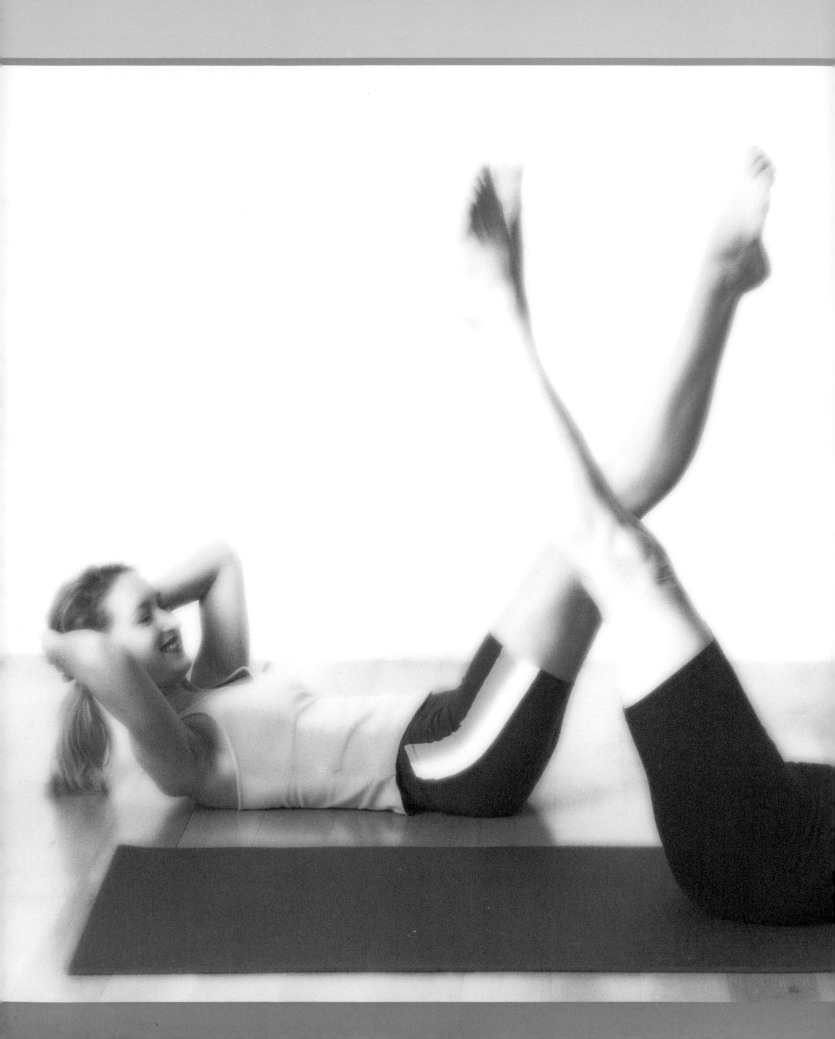

Introduction

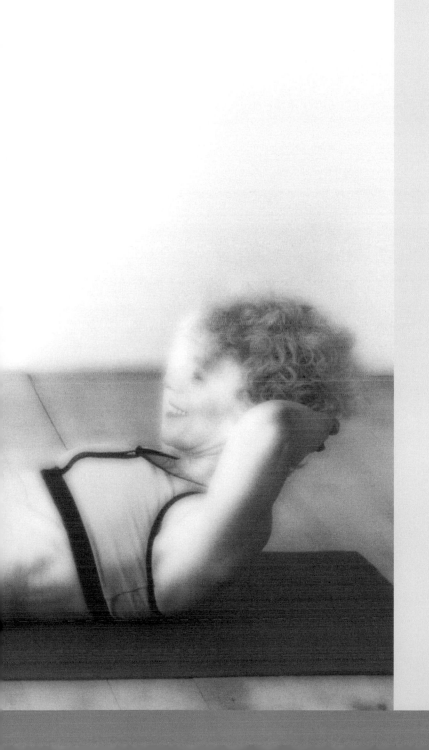

This book is the culmination of years of study and teaching the Pilates method. There are differing opinions among many Pilates practitioners about what technically can be considered a Pilates exercise. Some advocate leaving the method exactly as it was expounded by Joseph Pilates, while others believe it can be expanded to encompass exercises based on the principles of Pilates. This book portrays a wide variety of exercises which draw on both the original and newer exercise. I hope to achieve a harmony and fluidity between the different approaches to Pilates to help the reader understand fully the broad umbrella that Joseph Pilates work embodies today.

Joseph Hubertus Pilates (1880–1967)

Joseph Pilates was born near Dusseldorf, Germany, in 1880. As a small child he was sickly, with ailments such as asthma, rickets and rheumatic fever. He worked hard to overcome his symptoms through physical activities, including gymnastics, skiing and diving. He improved so much that by the time he was 14 years old, he was used as the model for anatomy charts. When Joseph Pilates was 31 he moved to England where he became a boxer, a circus performer and a self-defence trainer.

When the First World War broke out, Pilates was interned on the Isle of Man because of his German citizenship. During this time he worked in the prison hospital and began to develop equipment to aid bedridden patients. By rigging springs to the walls over the beds, patients' limbs could be attached to them and their muscles exercised without the need for full locomotion. These were the crude beginnings of one of the main apparatuses of Pilates – the Reformer. After the war, Pilates moved back to Germany and continued working on his fitness regime.

Joseph Pilates travelled to America in 1926, and it was during the journey across the Atlantic that he met his future wife, a nurse named Clara. Pilates set up his first studio at 939 Eighth Avenue, in New York. While little is known about the studio's early years, Pilates gained in popularity with the dance community. *Dance Magazine* reported in its February 1956 issue that virtually every dancer in New York, and certainly everyone who has studied at Jacob's Pillow between 1939 and 1951, had meekly submitted to the spirited instruction of Joe Pilates. Pilates documented his beliefs on health and exercise in a book called *Return to Life*. Outside the dancing community, however, little was known of Pilates during his lifetime. But then Pilates always used to say that his innovations were 50 years ahead of their time. Joseph Pilates died in 1967 at the age of 87.

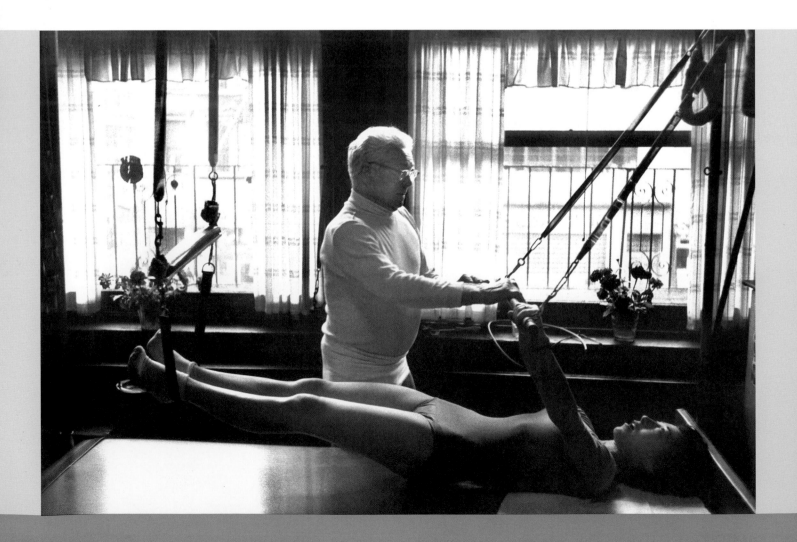

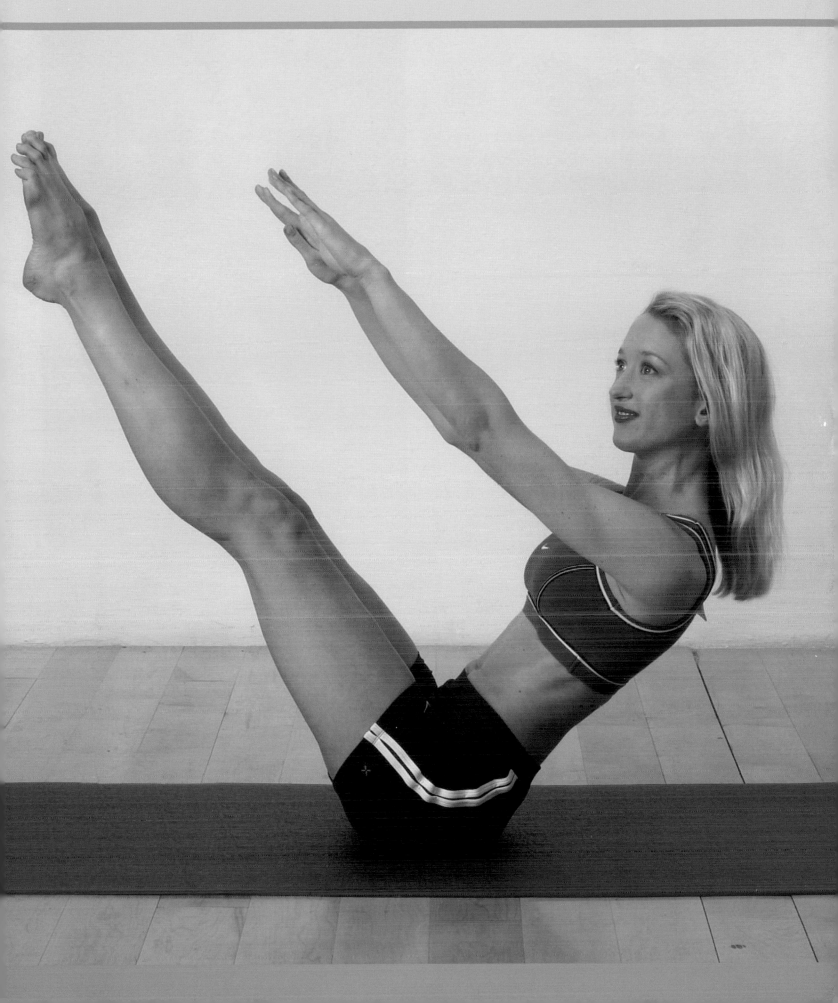

What is Pilates?

The Pilates method is a series of exercises created by Joseph Pilates to lengthen, strengthen and tone the body. Combining knowledge of Eastern and Western philosophies, the Pilates method focuses on core strength to assist in strengthening and stretching the entire body.

In Pilates, the mind and body are constantly working to develop supple, elongated muscles. This system combines stretching and strengthening with breathing and co-ordination to create a well-balanced body. Small muscle groups are brought into harmony with superficial ones. Posture improves and muscles become longer and leaner. There are very few repetitions of each exercise so the mind remains focused.

Dancers were initially drawn to Pilates because it made them stronger while keeping the body streamlined. However, Pilates exercises can be catered to the needs of each individual. Joseph Pilates based his work on mat exercises, but his innovative approach also used spring resistance in conjunction with anatomical opposition to achieve the desired results.

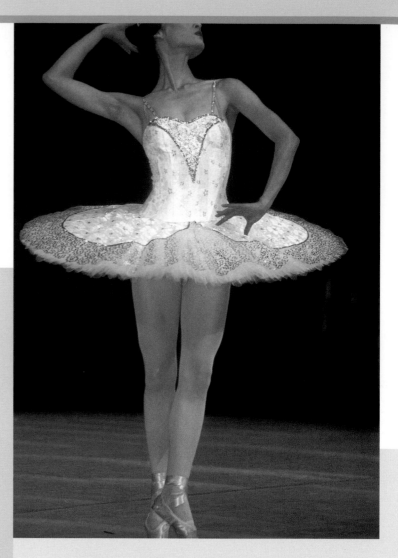

▲ Dancers use Pilates to strengthen and tone while still remaining supple.

Why Pilates?

Pilates can benefit anyone. It is for the young, the mature the disabled and the agile. It is unique because it adapts to suit the needs of the individual, and the variations are countless. A young dancer can do Pilates to avoid surgery and the injuries that come with over-use. A mature person can do Pilates exercises to improve posture, range of motion and locomotion. One 75-year-old client keeps coming back because he doesn't have pain getting in and out of taxis anymore! Pilates gives you the energy and flexibility to be more awake and alert throughout the day. Whether you have a few minutes or an hour to spare, Pilates can help centre and focus the mind and body. Everyone can benefit from exercises based upon the principles of Pilates.

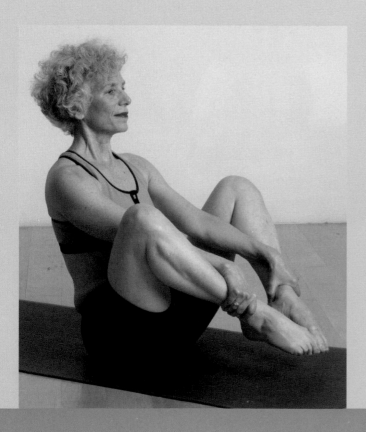

◄ Pilates is of benefit to anyone of any age.

Why the Pilates mat?

The fundamental key to Pilates is mat work. By doing the mat exercises daily, you can change the way you think, feel and move. Because there are few repetitions of each exercise, your mind remains constantly focused. Joseph Pilates also invented over 20 apparatuses in his lifetime, all of them to aid mat work. These machines offer resistance that makes performing the exercises easier than just using natural body weight. However, all of the exercise in this book can be done without the use of extra equipment.

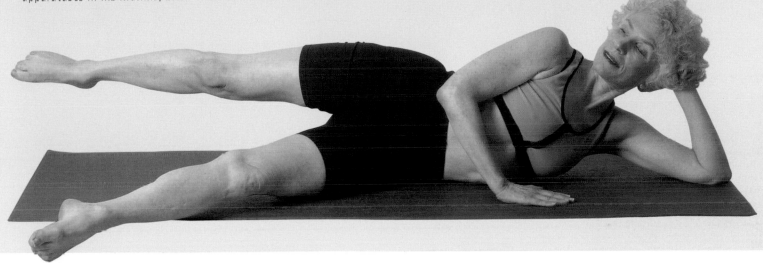

Why is it important to distinguish between the various methods?

Joseph Pilates taught a specific set of exercises in a specific order. There is debate in the Pilates world as to what can be considered a Pilates exercise. Different teachers might teach entirely different routines depending on where they studied. Personally, I believe that all these approaches are valid as long as they remain within the principles of Pilates. I also believe that the different variations and approaches work in harmony to create the results you want to achieve. Some of my clients only want to learn the original Pilates method. No problem! In this book, all of the exercises that were taught by Joseph Pilates are marked with (*). If you wish, you may follow only those exercises and sequences. However, I ask you not to dismiss the other exercises as there is much to learn if we are all open to it.

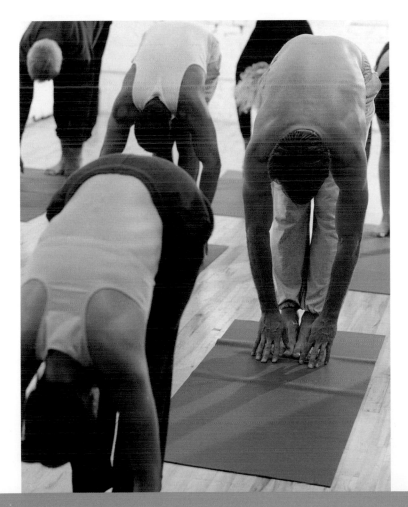

◄ Pilates can be taught in groups or individually.

Anatomy

A basic understanding of muscles and how they function is essential to any exercise regime. It is important to be able to visualise the muscles, or muscle groups, that are working in order to identify and isolate the areas that should be working. Pilates brings smaller muscles into harmony with larger ones. It is often said that Pilates makes you work muscles you never knew you had!

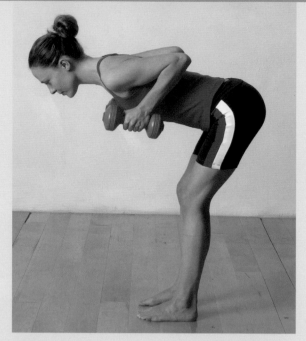

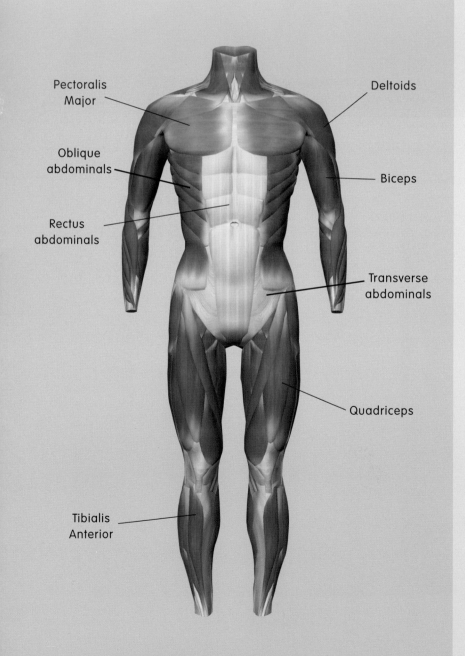

Pectoralis Major

Deltoids

Oblique abdominals

Biceps

Rectus abdominals

Transverse abdominals

Quadriceps

Tibialis Anterior

The triceps in these photos are acting as the synergists, while the biceps are relaxing, or acting as the antagonists.

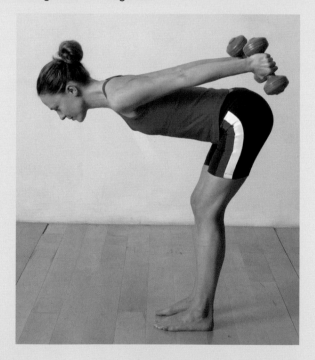

There are three types of muscles: cardiac, smooth and skeletal. Cardiac muscle is found only in the heart. Smooth muscle is involuntary and found in places such as the stomach and lining of the intestines. Skeletal muscle is voluntary and found in the muscles that we control consciously, such as the arms and legs. Pilates focuses on identifying and isolating the skeletal muscles.

Muscles consist of fibrous tissue surrounded by a connective sheath called fascia. Fascia elongates into dense connective tissue, known as tendon, which attaches muscles to bones. Each muscle attaches to two bones: one bone stays still, or fixed, and the other moves. The tendon that attaches to the bone that remains still is called the origin. The tendon that attaches to the bone that moves when the muscle contracts is called the insertion.

Usually, muscles contract in groups to create movement. When one set of muscles contracts, another set relaxes. The contracting muscles are called synergists, and the relaxing muscles antagonists. Depending on the movement, every muscle can be either a synergist or an antagonist. For example, the biceps bends the elbow joint (synergist) and the triceps relaxes to allow the elbow to bend (antagonist). Conversely, the triceps contracts to straighten the elbow joint (synergist) and the biceps relaxes (antagonist).

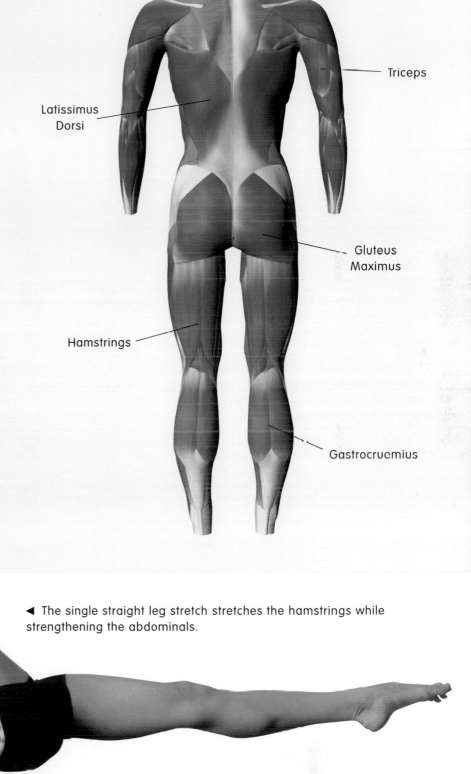

Trapezius

Levator Scapulae

Triceps

Latissimus Dorsi

Gluteus Maximus

Hamstrings

Gastrocruemius

◄ The single straight leg stretch stretches the hamstrings while strengthening the abdominals.

A word on posture

Most people barely notice in their daily lives how they sit, stand and walk. Yet how you present yourself to the world is usually a reflection of how you are feeling.

Have you ever noticed someone walking with a sunken chest, droopy shoulders and eyes on the ground and thought, 'Cheer up! Life's not that bad'? Have you ever stood tall, shoulders open, eyes up, and noticed you felt great? Besides making you feeling better, correct posture creates less wear and tear on the spine over time.

Ideal posture is when the highest point of the ear is in line with the centre of the shoulder, which in turn is in line with the hip. Try standing in front of a mirror. Notice if your shoulders are rounding forwards. Now turn your thumbs out and notice if the shoulders open slightly. Try and keep the shoulders open, and relax your thumbs. Now turn sideways and look in the mirror. See if the top of the ear is in line with the centre of the shoulder, which is in line with the hip. Think of lengthening through the top of the head and extending energy through the feet to the floor. Now for the hard part – make it look natural!

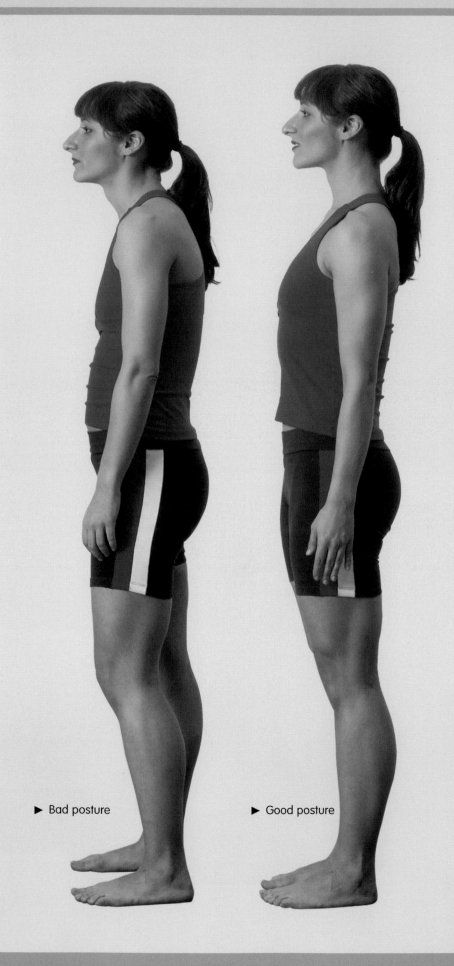

▶ Bad posture   ▶ Good posture

Pilates lingo

Pilates lingo refers to the commonly used terms that you will hear throughout a Pilates session. Pilates lingo, together with Pilates principles, are the building blocks for all Pilates exercises.

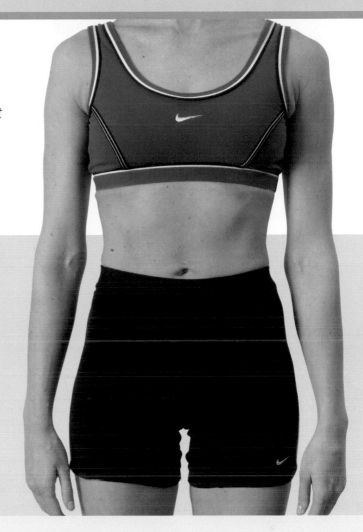

The powerhouse

Joseph Pilates created this concept to refer to the muscles of the abdominals, lower back and buttocks. He believed that more efficient movement could be achieved if it originated from the powerhouse. This is just one of the concepts that makes Pilates a unique and dynamic form of exercise.

Elongated feet

The feet in Pilates are relaxed and long, unless otherwise stated. The foot extends and lengthens through space with the toes relaxed. A good rule of thumb is that someone could come up and wiggle your toes and they would be relaxed, not stiff.

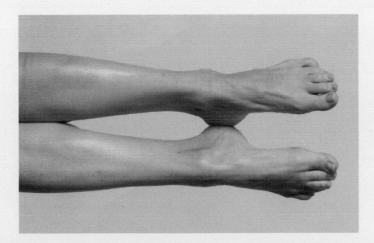

1 Correct – feet are long and relaxed.

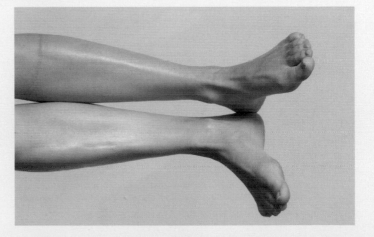

2 Incorrect – feet are not extending through space.

Extension

Every movement in Pilates involves extending through space. Think of energy extending beyond your extremities and feel your head lengthening away from your tailbone. Think of energy going down through your heels and fingertips. As you perform the exercises, lengthen through space, trying to extend your body without being rigid.

1 No extension throughout the body.

2 Energy lengthening through the extremities.

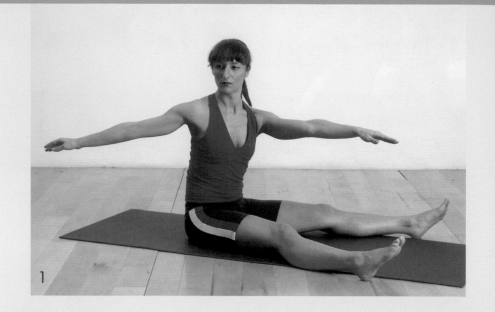

1

2

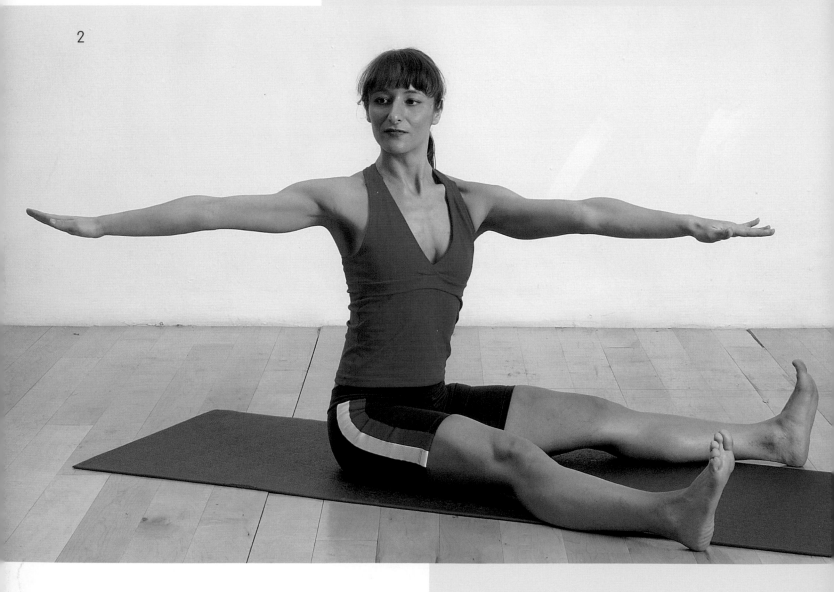

Neutral spine

The concept of the neutral spine has evolved since Joseph Pilates' death, but it is taught so regularly as part of the Pilates method that it must be incorporated. Due to advances in science and exercise, it is now considered integral to the system. Neutral spine refers to the natural alignment of the curvature of the spine. While this is easy to find standing up, it is much more difficult lying down. The easiest way is to lie on your back with your knees bent and your feet hip-width apart. Roll the tailbone up so that the hips are tucking under. Then roll the pelvis back so that you are arching. Do this a few times until you can find the centre of these two movements. This is what is considered neutral spine.

Pelvic floor

Although the term 'pelvic floor' was not used, the concept was part of the original Pilates system. If you pull in your powerhouse and engage your deep transverse abdominus, then your pelvic floor muscles engage. The pelvic floor muscles are a light web of muscles that control the dispersal of waste products from the body. The easiest way to find these muscles is to pretend you need to use the loo! You will feel a slight lifting up of the muscles underneath your pelvis. Try to think of these muscles contracting as part of the girdle of strength. Another way to find your pelvic floor muscles is to suck your thumb. Bizarre but true!

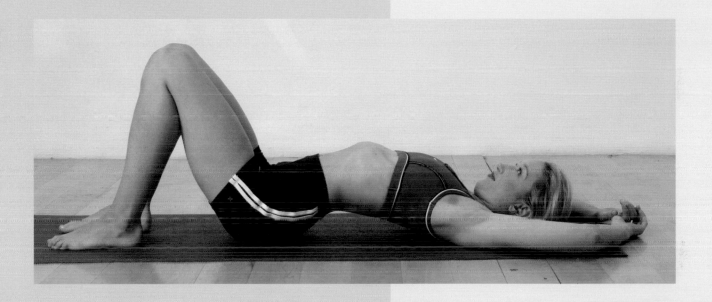

▲ Neutral spine - incorrect. Ribs are out and the back is arched.

▶ Neutral spine - correct. Note the slight natural curve in the spine.

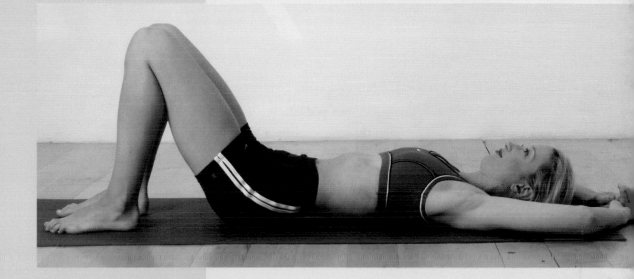

Pilates principles

Pilates principles are the fundamentals of all Pilates exercises. While performing each exercise, be aware of your concentration, control, centring, flow, precision and breath. They are the framework within which all movements should be executed.

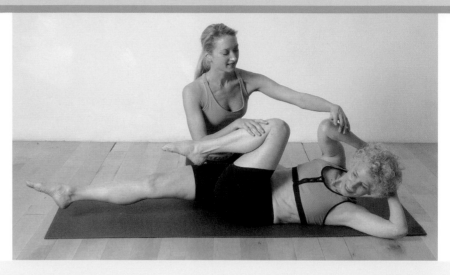

▲ The criss cross strengthens the obliques.

Concentration

'Concentrate on the correct movements each time you exercise, lest you do them improperly and thus lose all the vital benefits of their value.'
Joseph Pilates

Pilates changes the way you think, move and feel. The mind cannot wander to your shopping list while the body performs the movements. Pilates is about being present in the moment. By focusing on isolation and control of various muscle groups, it forces you to be present. It enhances awareness of the body, how it moves, and your control of it. Because there are so many aspects to think about, and so few repetitions of each exercise, the mind must constantly focus on the task at hand.

Control

In your daily life you create repetitive patterns of movement. Pilates changes your awareness of your body by bringing these repetitive movements under your conscious control. How often do you stand slouched over the sink brushing your teeth? By creating awareness of posture through specific exercises you become more conscious of everyday activities. Think about doing one hundred jumping jacks. By the time you have finished, you probably have no idea if your feet are parallel, your hips are square, your shoulders are down, and your abdominals are pulled in. Not so in Pilates! Every movement in Pilates requires the use of conscious control. Nothing is done in a haphazard way.

▶ The child's pose is a wonderful stretch for the spine.

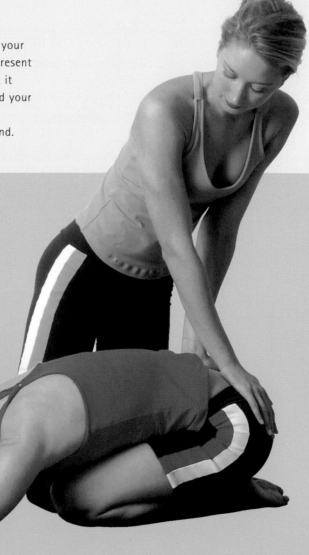

▶ The cat aids articulation of the spine.

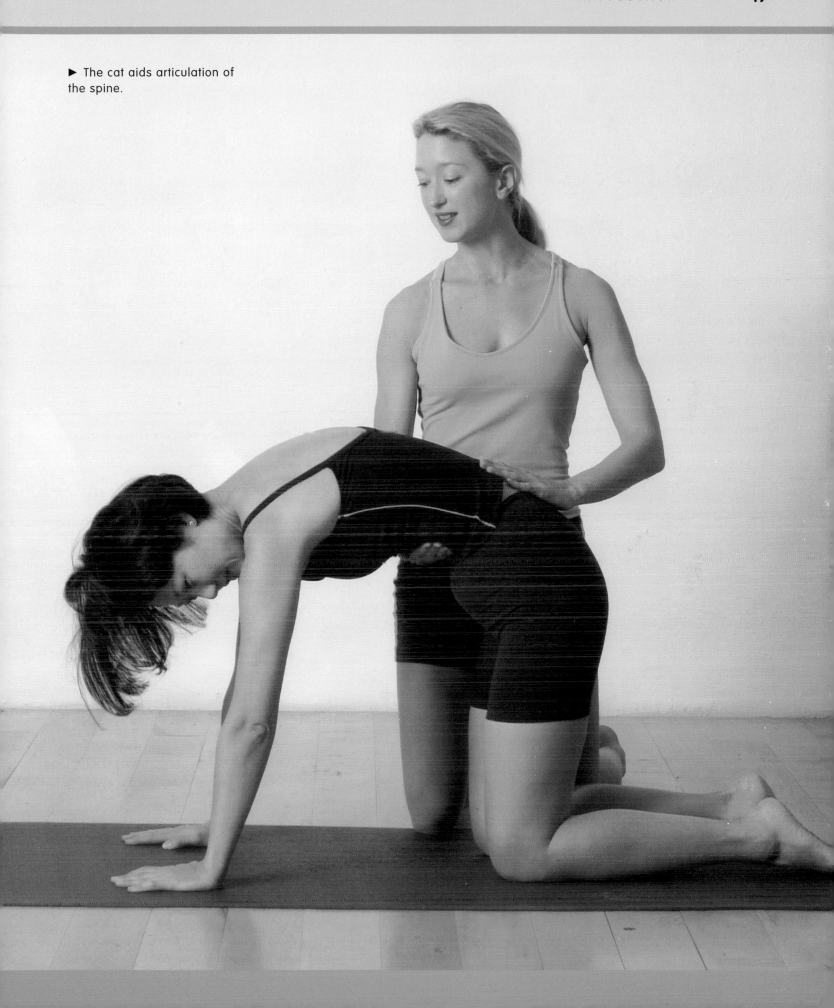

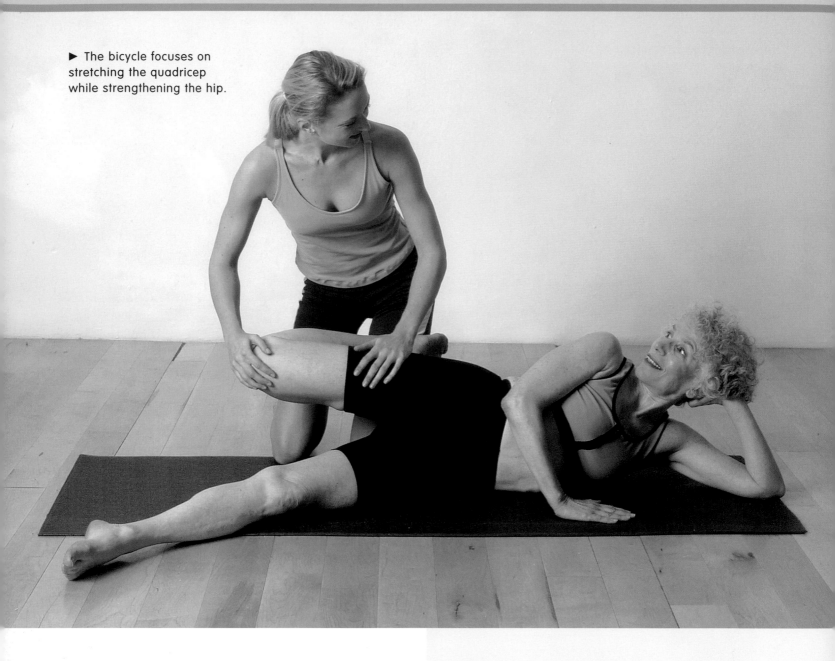

▶ The bicycle focuses on stretching the quadricep while strengthening the hip.

Centring

Joseph Pilates called the girdle of strength the powerhouse. Today, it is commonly called core stability. While core stability is a new term on the exercise front, the concept of movement originating from the centre is not. The muscles of the stomach, lower back, pelvic floor and bottom all come together to initiate outward movement. If you are doing an arm movement, or a leg movement, think of it coming from your centre. Imagine picking up a large box off the floor. If you bend over at the hips with straight legs, the pressure goes immediately into the lower back. If you bend your knees and pull the stomach in, the weight of the box does not affect the back. That's because you are moving from your centre!

Flow

Flow of movement is integral to the Pilates method. Each exercise has a rhythmic and dynamic quality, with a natural grace and flow to the movements. If it feels choppy and awkward then its not Pilates! In the original method, exercises are performed in a specific sequence with specific transitions in-between. These transitions are choreographed much in the same way as a dance is choreographed. The transitions are designed so that each movement flows gracefully into the next. It should not be apparent where one exercise stops and the next begins.

Precision

Joseph Pilates believed in efficiency of movement. Each exercise should be performed as correctly as possible while staying within your frame of strength or control. Movements should not be allowed to go beyond your range of motion.

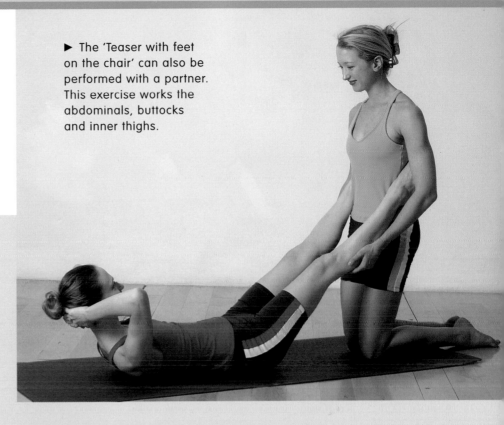

▶ The 'Teaser with feet on the chair' can also be performed with a partner. This exercise works the abdominals, buttocks and inner thighs.

Breath

Breath is the very essence of life. Without oxygen, we cannot live. Yet most of us go through life without consciously thinking of how we are breathing. Pilates brings conscious movement – such as the rise and fall of the rib cage as you inhale and exhale – to the surface. Each movement in Pilates corresponds to specific breathing patterns.

Pilates retrains the body to focus on how and when you breathe. The breath is called lateral breathing or thoracic breathing. Think of inhaling into the back and sides of the rib cage. Place your hands on the sides of the rib cage. Inhale and feel the ribs expand as your lungs fill with oxygen. Exhale and fell the ribs soften as the lungs collapse. Repeat this exercise a few times, consciously thinking of the movement of your breath.

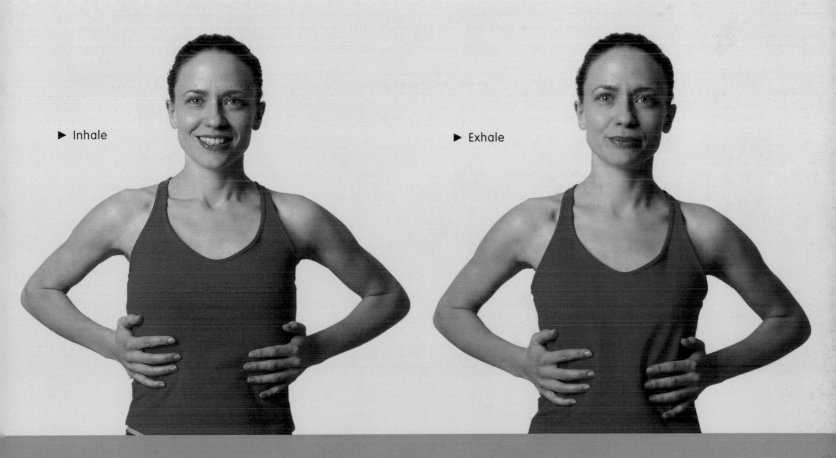

▶ Inhale

▶ Exhale

Pilates basics

What should I wear?

Wear loose, comfortable clothing – anything that you feel able to move in freely. Avoid wearing any item of clothing with zippers or belts as these will get in the way of the exercises. Pilates is done barefoot or in socks, with no shoes. Shoes inhibit the movements of the feet and add extra weight.

What do I need to get started?

Find a place where you can move without hitting anything. You might need a couple of pillows with different degrees of firmness. If you have some weights, great! Pilates does not require very heavy weights. Women need weights no heavier than 2kg/5lb, and men no heavier than 3kg/7lb. You will also need a firm chair on which you can sit with your legs bent with the knee at a right angle.

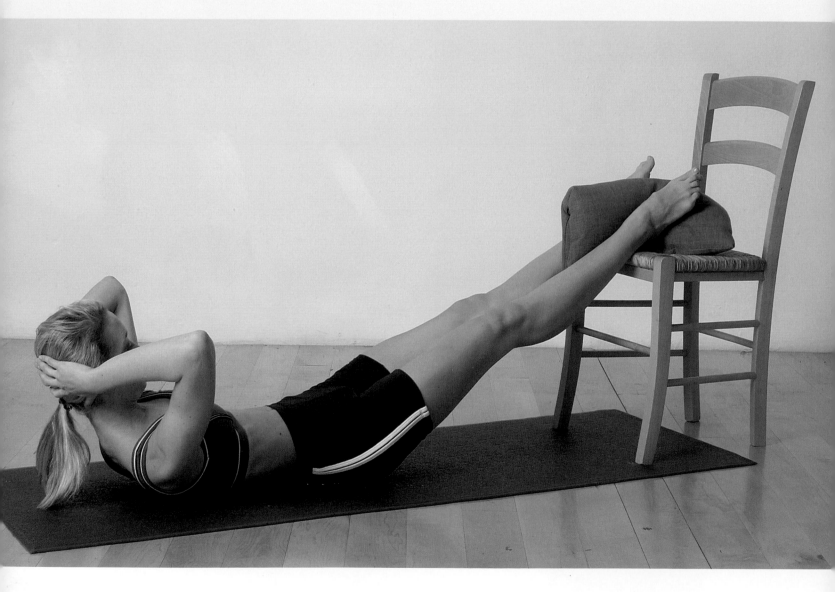

How to use this book

This book is divided into three sections. The Beginners' section teaches you correct posture and how to isolate your muscles. Isolation is important because it brings the smaller muscle groups into harmony with larger muscle groups. Please do not skip this section because the exercises look easy. They are designed to help you break down movements so that you can piece them together in later exercises. The Intermediate exercises help you to take the isolations and start putting them together. By slowly adding each of the isolations, total control of the whole body can be achieved. The Advanced section is the original Pilates mat as Joseph Pilates used to teach it. This section takes time to master effectively.

Each section begins with a quick reference guide showing the exercises which follow. At the end of each section is a 15-minute workout intended as a shorter Pilates session. Some exercises have additional modifications or challenges; please refer to them if you are feeling either overly challenged or under-stretched. Move on to the next section only when you have mastered the exercises in the previous section.

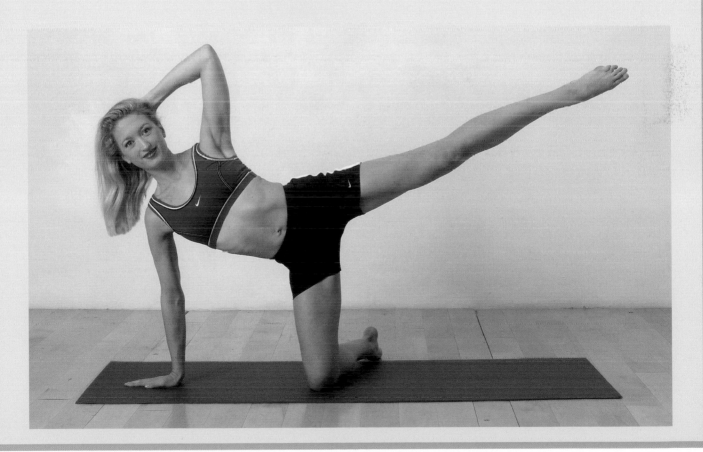

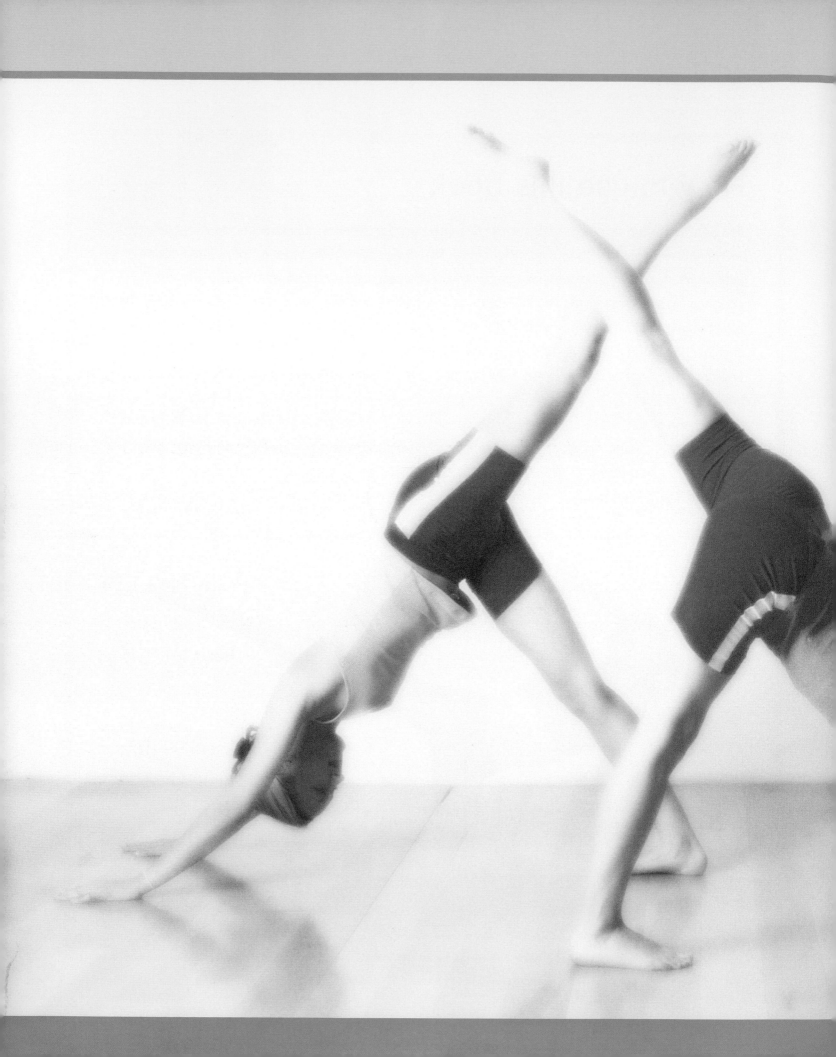

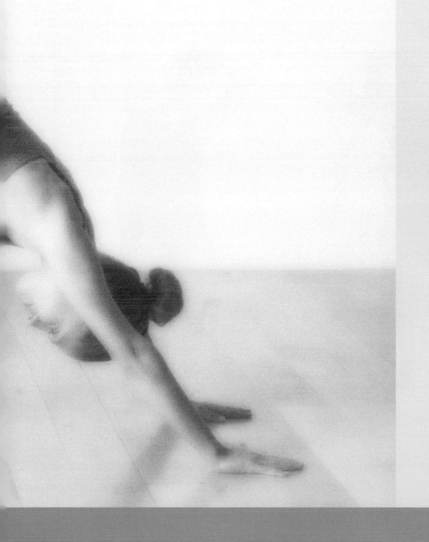

Beginners

'As small bricks are employed to build large buildings, so the development of small muscles helps to develop large muscles and, ultimately, your entire body.'

Joseph Pilates

'I started Pilates at the age of 75. The doctor asked why I bothered as I had survived so long without it. I replied that I could no longer get in and out of London taxis without hauling myself up! After three months of Pilates training, I can now use a taxi like a 21-year-old.'

Brian Sandalson

Introduction

This first section consists of Pilates-based exercises. Most of these exercises are designed by Alan Herdman in London, and they have been taught by him for over 30 years.

The exercises in this section help you to identify how to isolate specific muscles so that you can put all of the isolations together in the later sections. It is important to learn how to isolate various muscles in order to bring the body into balance. Larger muscles have a tendency to take over while smaller muscle groups become weaker, putting the body out of alignment. By bringing smaller muscle groups into harmony with larger muscle groups, more efficiency of movement can be achieved. The sequence of these exercises is designed to stretch and strengthen various muscle groups.

The first nine exercises are postural exercises and are performed sitting in a chair. Postural exercises improve awareness and body alignment. Use a firm chair on which you can sit with your legs bent at the knee at a right angle.

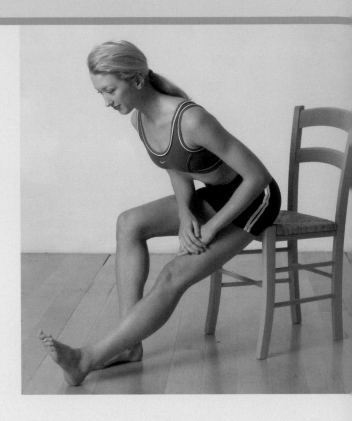

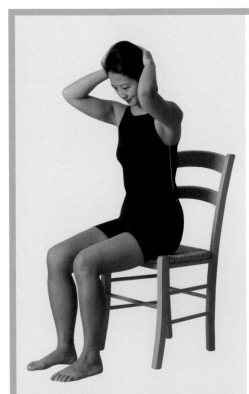

1. Neck Stretch Front. See page 30.

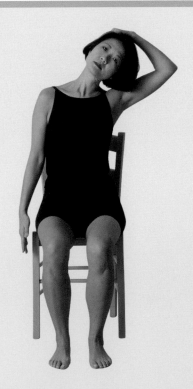

2. Neck Stretches Side. See page 32.

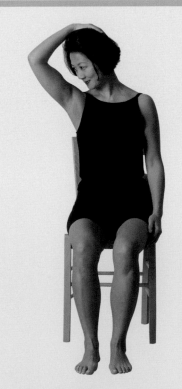

3. Neck Stretches on the Diagonal. See page 34.

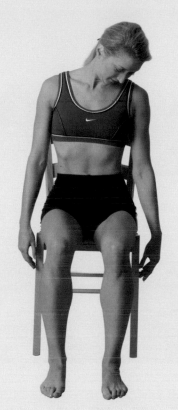

4. Head Circles. See page 36.

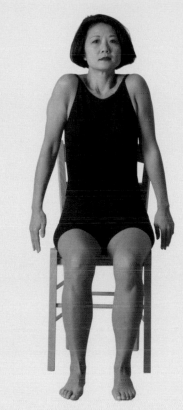

5. Shoulder Shrugs. See page 38.

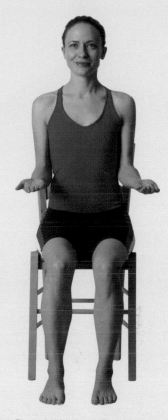

6. Dumb Waiter. See page 40.

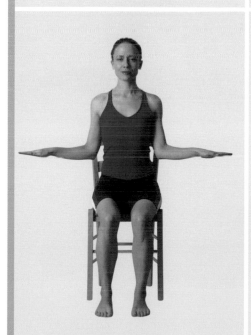

7 Opening. See page 42.

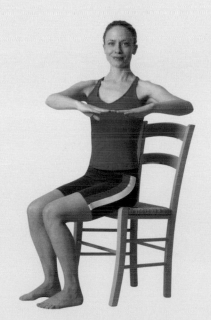

8. Beginner's Twist.
See page 44.

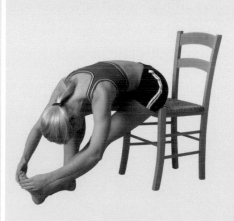

9. Hamstring Stretch Sitting.
See page 46.

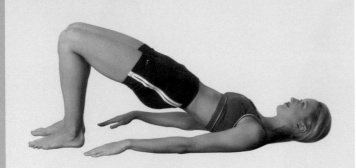

10. Pelvic Curl. See page 48.

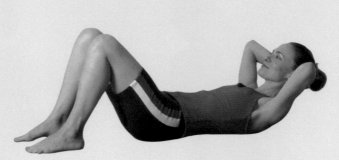

11. Abdominals . See page 50.

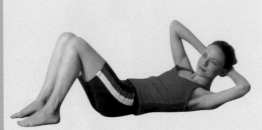

12. Obliques. See page 52.

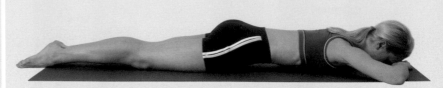

13. Buttocks Squeeze. See page 54.

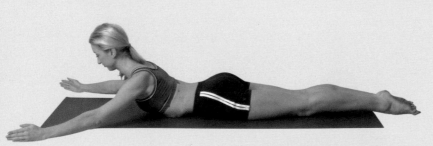

14. Shoulder Blades. See page 55.

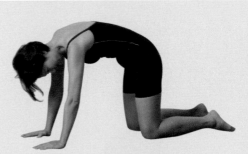

15. Cat. See page 56.

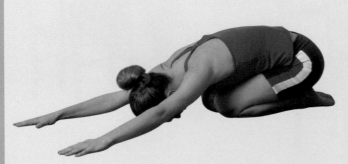

16. Child's Pose. See page 58.

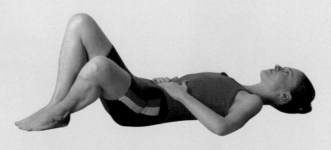

17. Abdominal Isolation. See page 59.

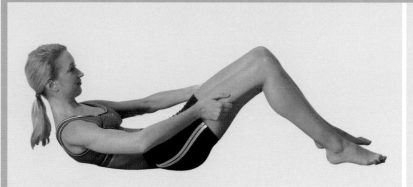

18. Abdominals with Arm Extension. See page 60.

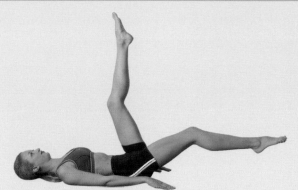

19. Single Leg Lifts. See page 62.

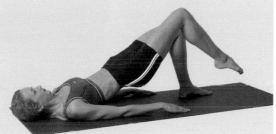

20. Pelvic Curls with Leg Lifts. See page 64.

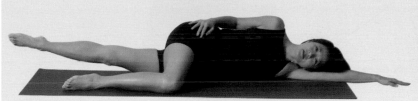

21. Inner Thigh. See page 66.

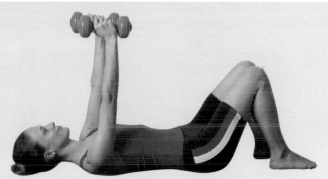

22. Triceps. See page 67.

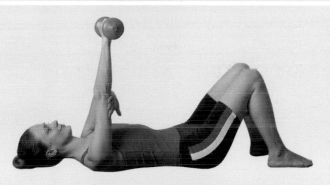

23. Karate Chops. See page 68.

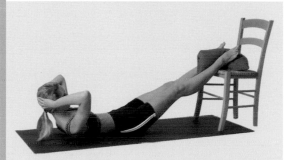

24. Teaser with Feet on Chair. See page 69.

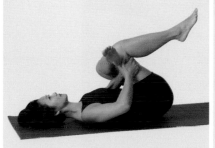

25. Hip Stretch 1. See page 70.

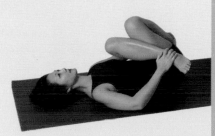

26. Hip Stretch 2. See page 71.

Neck Stretch Front

The Neck Stretch Front is a wonderful warm-up exercise designed to stretch the back of the neck.

1 Sit on the front edge of a chair. Place your feet flat on the floor with your legs parallel and hip-width apart.

2

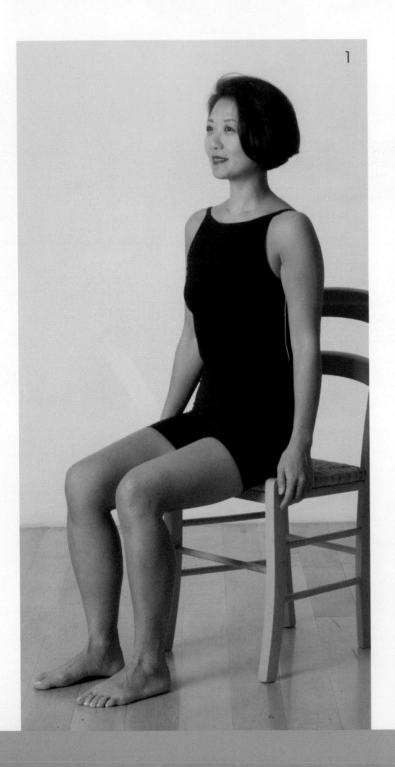

1

2 Lace your fingers and place the hands directly behind your head with the elbows to the side. Inhale to prepare.

3

3 As you exhale, slowly bring the head and elbows forwards while lengthening through the back of the neck. Keep the back in a neutral sitting position. Relax the weight of the arms on to the back of the head without pulling.

4 Stay in this position, inhaling and exhaling for three deep breaths.

5 Relax and come back to the centre.

Key Points:

- Keep the knees and feet hip-width apart.

- Keep the navel into the spine and breathe through the sides and back of the ribs.

- Do not pull with the arms; this can create too much tension and pressure on the back of the neck

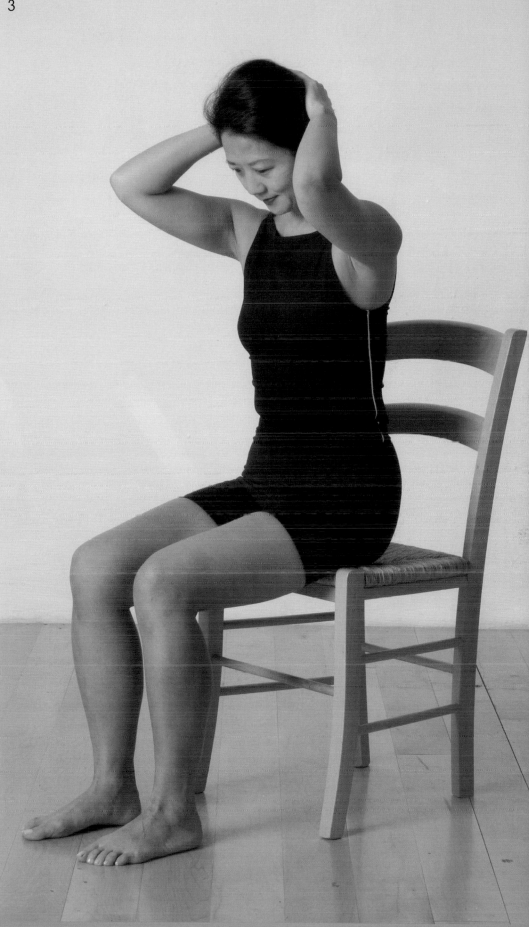

Neck Stretches Side

Neck Stretches Side targets the neck muscles on the opposite side of the neck from the direction in which you are leaning.

1

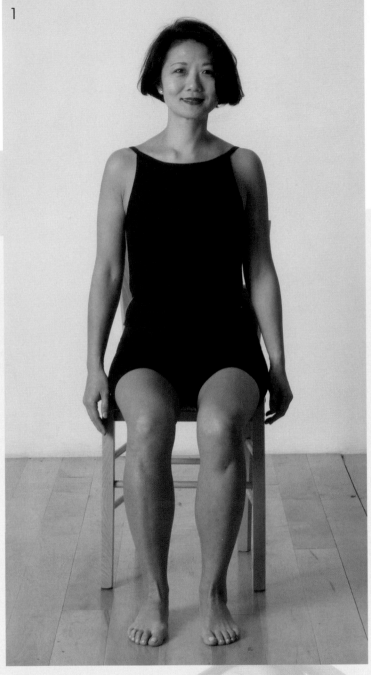

1 Sit on the front edge of a chair. Your feet should be parallel and the legs hip-width apart.

2

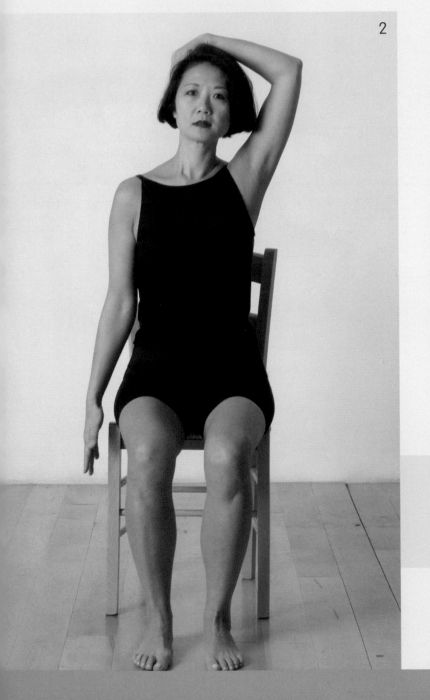

2 Looking straight ahead, place your left arm over the top of your head and your left hand on your right ear. Your right arm should be extending down to the floor. Inhale to prepare.

3

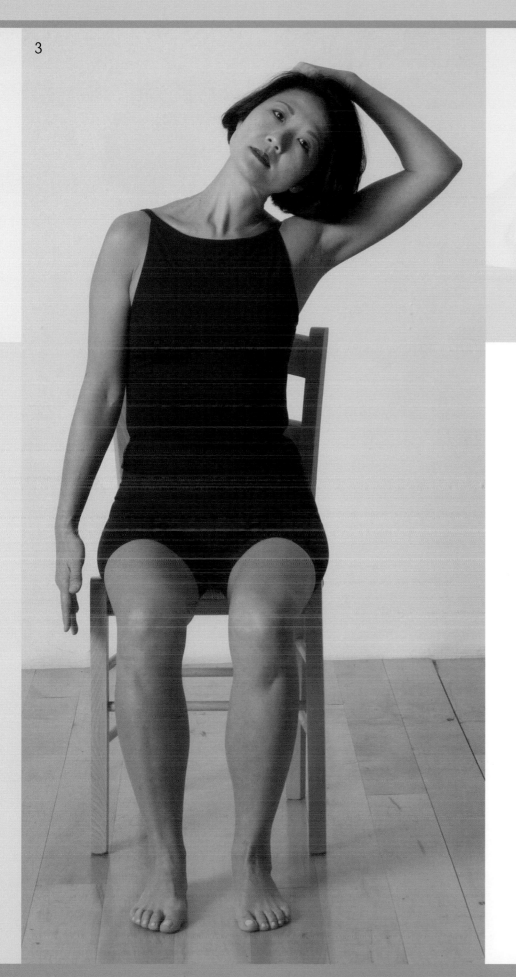

3 As you exhale, tilt your head to the left, while envisioning your left ear going towards your left shoulder. Stay in this position for three deep breaths.

4 Come back to the starting position.

5 Repeat on the other side.

Key Points:

- Keep the knees and feet hip-width apart.

- Keep the navel into the spine and breathe through the sides and back of the ribs.

- Keep the shoulders relaxed and even the whole time.

- Do not pull with the arms; this can create too much tension and pressure on the back of the neck.

Neck Stretches on the Diagonal

Neck Stretches on the Diagonal releases the muscles on the opposite side of the back of the neck.

1 Sit on the front edge of a chair. Your feet should be flat on the ground, parallel to each other and hip-width apart. The head begins looking forwards in a neutral position, in line with the spine. Turn the head to the right, so that your head is approximately 45 degrees.

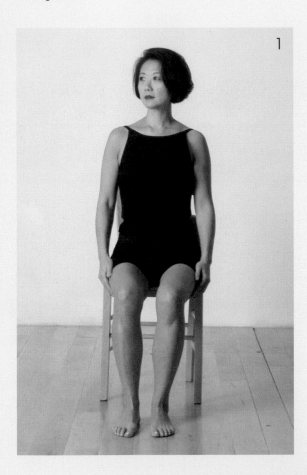

1

2 Take the right arm up and over your head and place the hand directly behind your head. Your left arm should be relaxed down by your side. You should be looking into your elbow. Inhale to prepare.

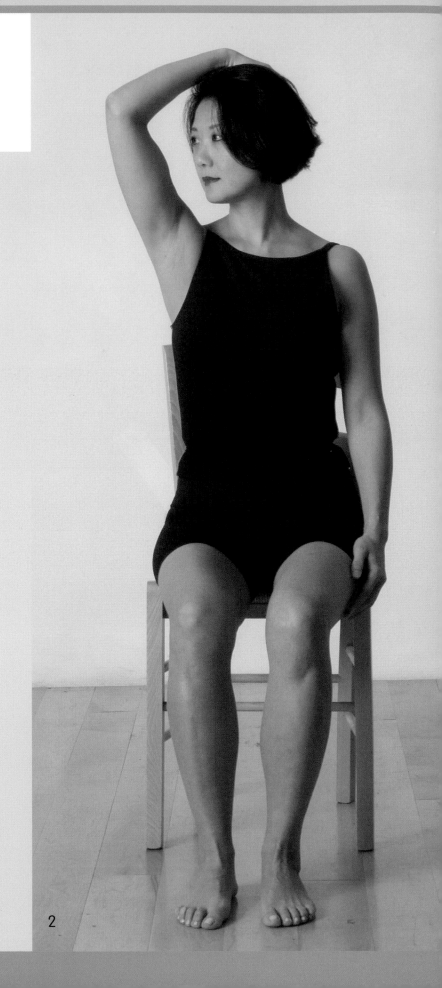

2

3 Exhale and drop your chin down, so that you feel a stretch in the opposite side of the neck. Stay in this position for three deep breaths.

4 Come back to the centre, and repeat the whole movement to the left.

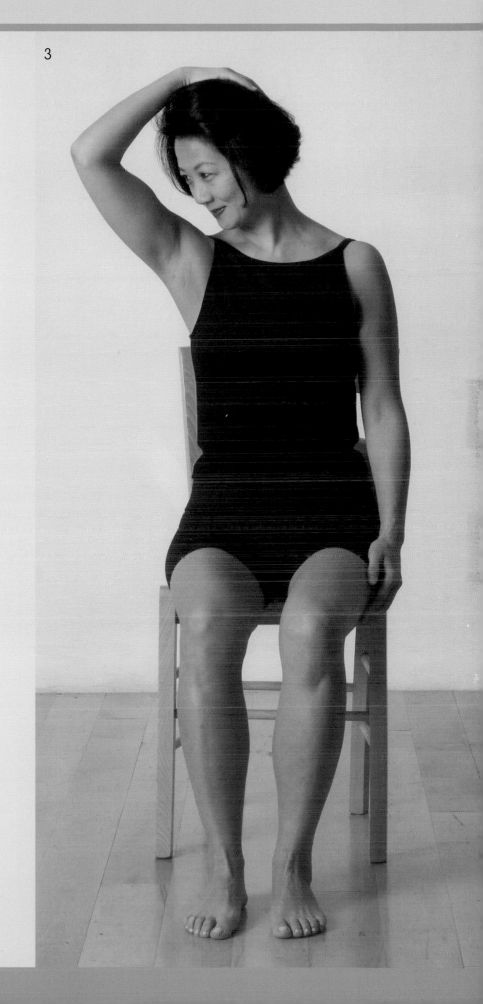

3

Key Points:

- Keep the knees and feet hip-width apart.

- Keep the navel into the spine and breathe through the sides and back of the ribs.

- Keep the shoulders relaxed and even the whole time.

- Do not to pull with the arms; this can create too much tension and pressure on the back of the neck.

Head Circles

Head Circles release tension in the muscles in the back of the neck.

1 Sitting on the front edge of a chair, place your feet flat on the floor and hip-width apart. Inhale as you lengthen your head towards the ceiling.

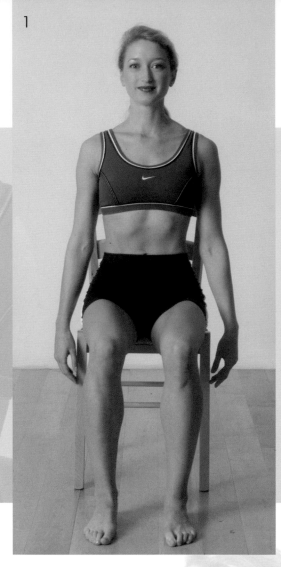

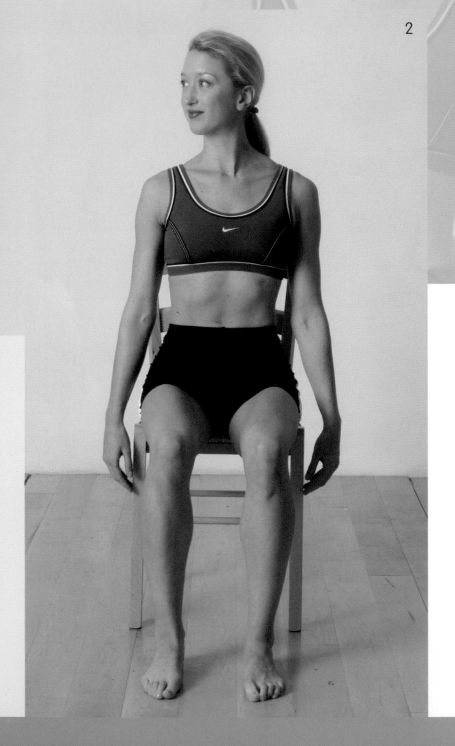

2 As you exhale, slowly look over your right shoulder.

3

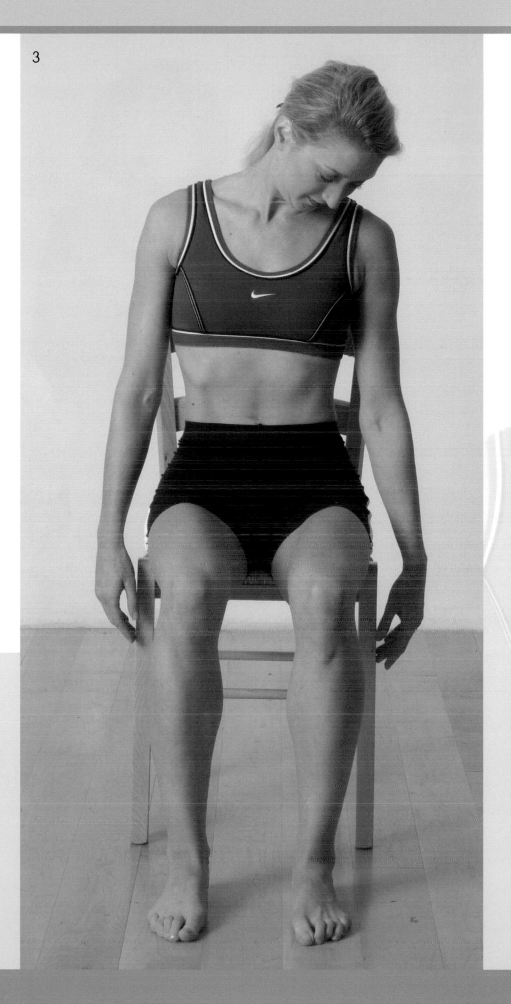

3 Drop the chin down towards your right, circle the head forwards and down until the chin is all the way over towards your left shoulder. Inhale to come back to centre.

4 Immediately reverse. Exhale looking over your left shoulder; drop your chin down and forwards, circling your head to the right.

5 Repeat the whole exercise four times.

Key Points:

- Keep the knees and feet hip-width apart.

- Keep the navel into the spine and breathe through the sides and back of the ribs.

- Keep the shoulders relaxed and even the whole time.

Shoulder Shrugs

Shoulder Shrugs is a great warm-up exercise to relax the shoulders and engage the back.

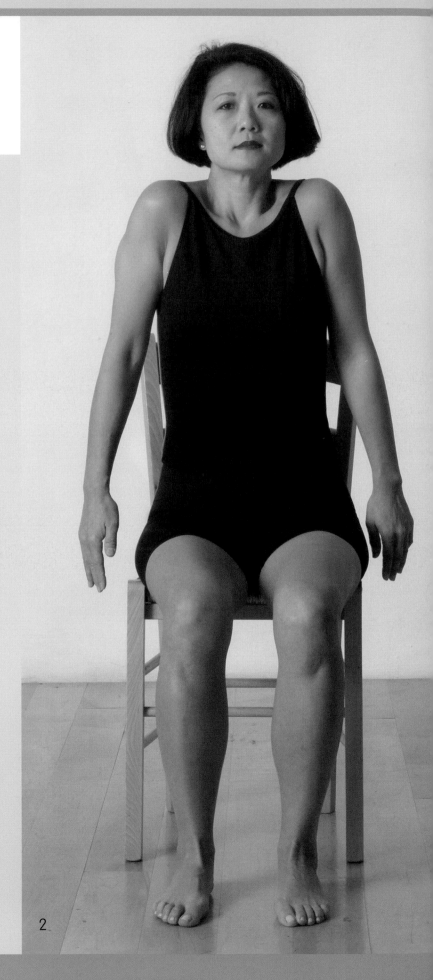

1 Sit on a chair with your feet hip-width apart and your knees parallel. Make sure you are sitting up on your seat bones and your head is lengthening to the ceiling with your arms relaxed by your sides.

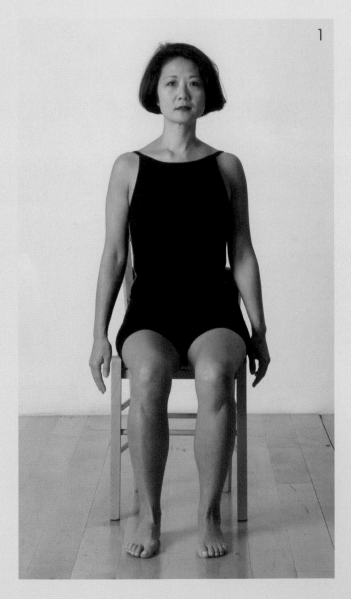

2 As you inhale, raise your shoulders up to your ears.

3

3 As you exhale, relax your shoulders and press your fingertips down to the ground and back behind you. Your palms should be facing backwards.

4 When you need to inhale, relax your hands and raise your shoulders up to your ears again.

5 Repeat the whole exercise ten times.

Key Points:

- Make sure your chest stays open and wide as your hands pull down and back.

- Lengthen the top of your head to the ceiling.

- Keep the navel pulling into the spine and breathe through the sides and back of the ribs.

- Keep the feet and knees hip-width apart.

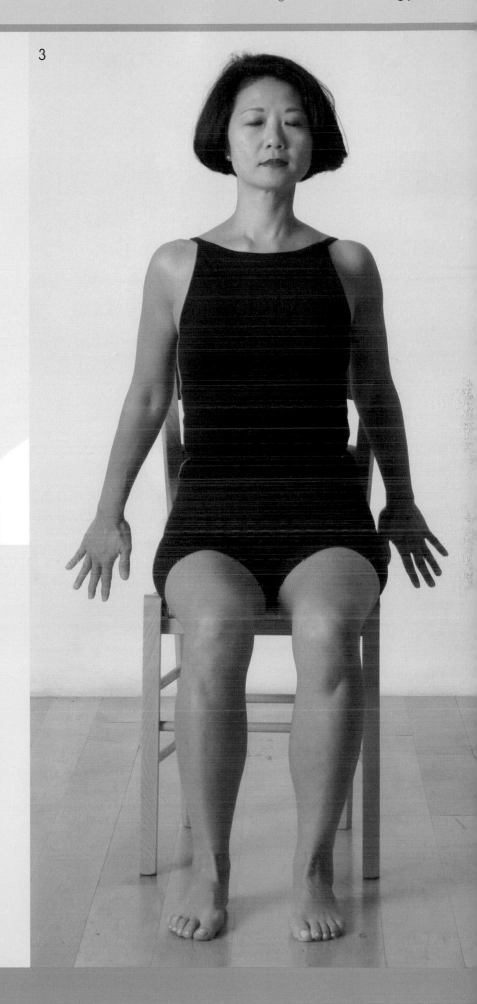

Dumb Waiter

The Dumb Waiter focuses on posture. Think of the alignment of your head and shoulders as you work on maintaining your arms in the shoulder socket.

1 Sit in a chair with your feet hip-width apart and your knees parallel to each other.

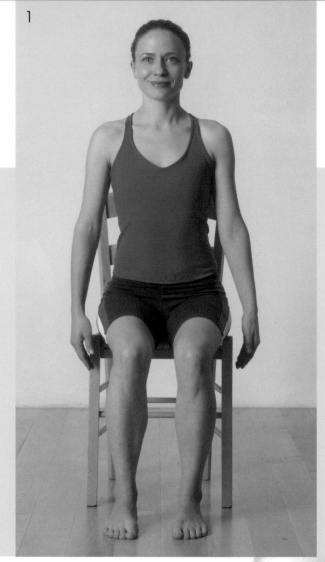

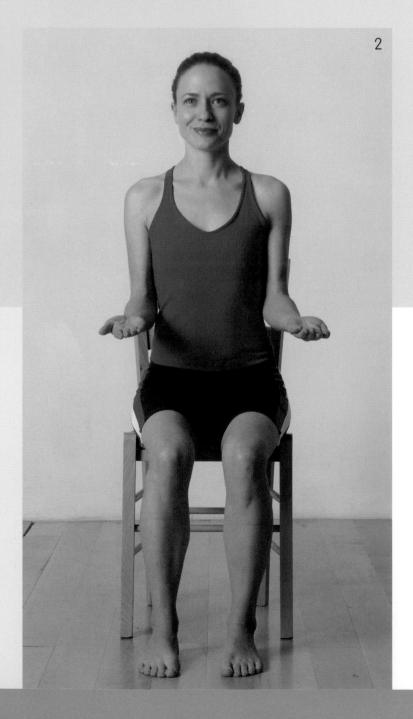

2 Lengthen your head towards the ceiling. Bend your arms at right angles with the palms facing upwards. Keep your elbows into the ribcage at all times. Inhale to prepare.

3 As you exhale, bring your forearms and hands to the sides.

4 As you inhale, bring the hands back to the original position. Keep the shoulders as open as possible.

5 Repeat ten times.

3

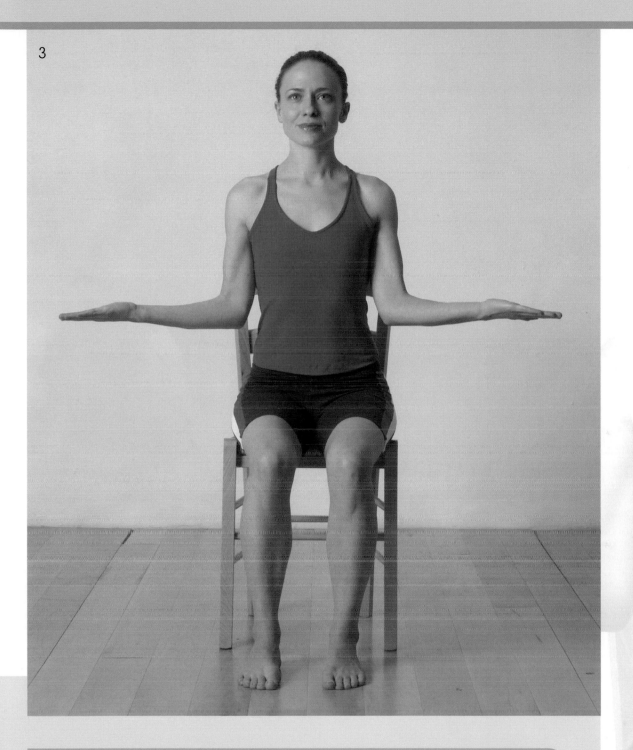

Key Points:

- Make sure the head does not go forwards as the hands reach to your sides.

- Keep the shoulder cuff open as you bring your hands back to the centre.

- Keep the navel into the spine and breathe through the sides and back of the ribs.

- Keep the feet and knees hip-width apart.

- Lengthen the top of the head towards the ceiling.

Opening

The Opening works on initiating arm movement with the muscles around the shoulder blades rather than with the arm itself. Focus on feeling the initiation of the movement from the shoulder blades, while engaging the abdominals.

1 Sit on a chair with your feet hip-width apart and your knees parallel to each other.

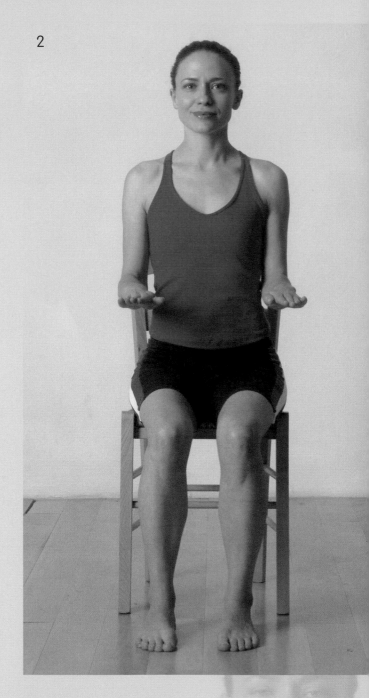

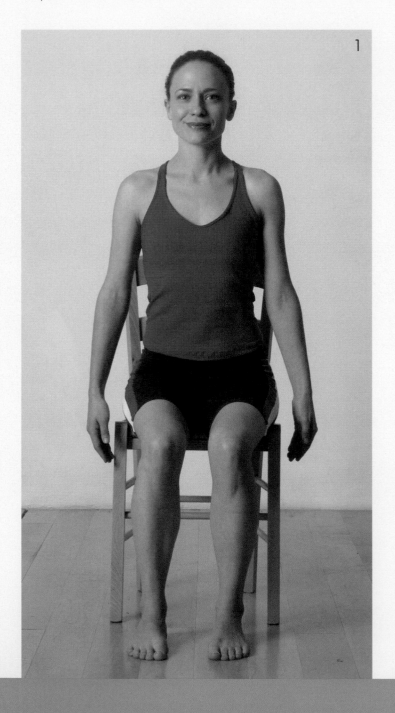

2 Bend your arms at right angles, with your elbows into your ribs and your palms facing downwards. Inhale to prepare.

3   As you exhale, initiate the arms moving to the sides by pulling your shoulder blades back and together.

4   Inhale, releasing the shoulder blades and letting your arms float back to the original position.

5   Repeat ten times.

Key Points:

- Make sure the elbows touch your ribcage the whole time on this exercise.

- Keep the shoulder cuff open as you bring your hands back to the centre.

- Keep the navel into the spine and breathe through the sides and back of the ribs.

- Keep the feet and knees hip-width apart.

- Lengthen the top of the head towards the ceiling.

- Make sure the head does not go forwards as the hands reach to your sides.

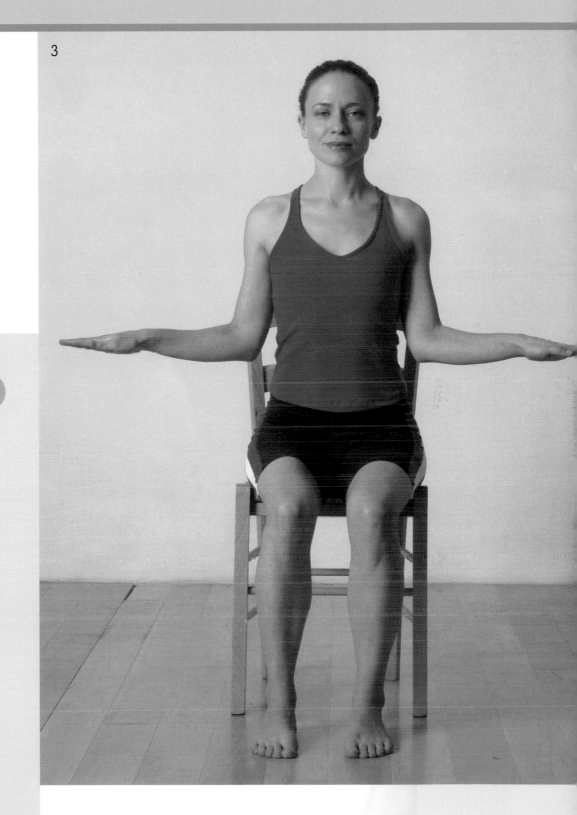

3

Beginner's Twist

The Beginner's Twist is designed for mobility, length of the spine and posture. Focus on isolating the muscles around your shoulder blades while lengthening through the top of your head and keeping the shoulders relaxed.

1 Sit with your feet hip-width apart and your knees parallel to each other.

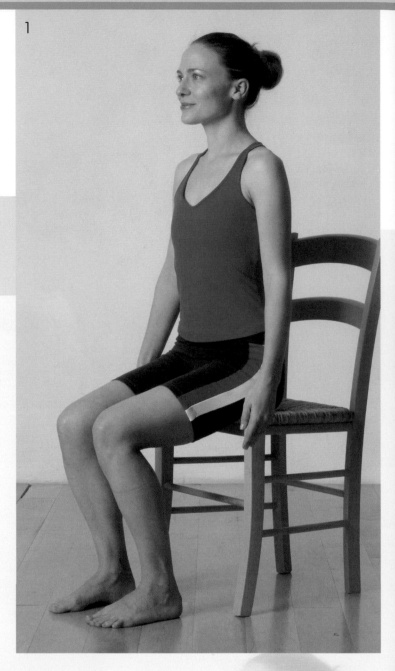

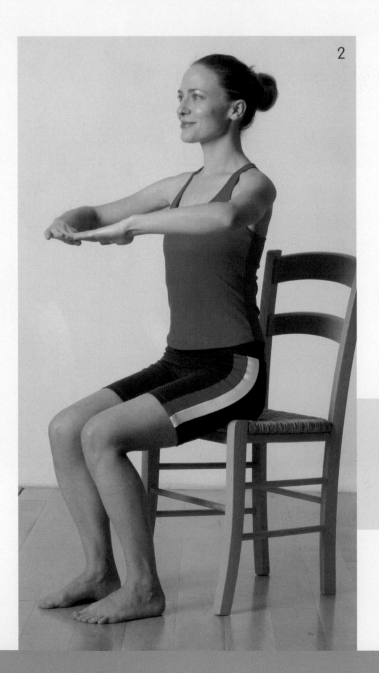

2 Place your fingertips together and your elbows out to the sides so that your arms are forming a circle. Place your hands in front of you in front of your chest. Think of dropping your shoulder blades down and lifting your head to the ceiling. Inhale to prepare.

3

3 As you exhale, pull the left shoulder blade down as you turn your upper torso towards the left, leaving the hands in front of the chest at all times. Think of pulling your right shoulder downwards while keeping both shoulders even.

4 Inhale back to the centre.

5 As you take your second exhale, start by pulling the right shoulder blade down and moving towards the right.

6 Inhale to come back to the centre.

7 Repeat four times each side.

Key Points:

- Keep the shoulder blades pulling down the back.

- Keep the feet and knees hip-width apart.

- Keep the head lengthening towards the ceiling.

- Make sure the shoulders stay even and the hips do not twist or move.

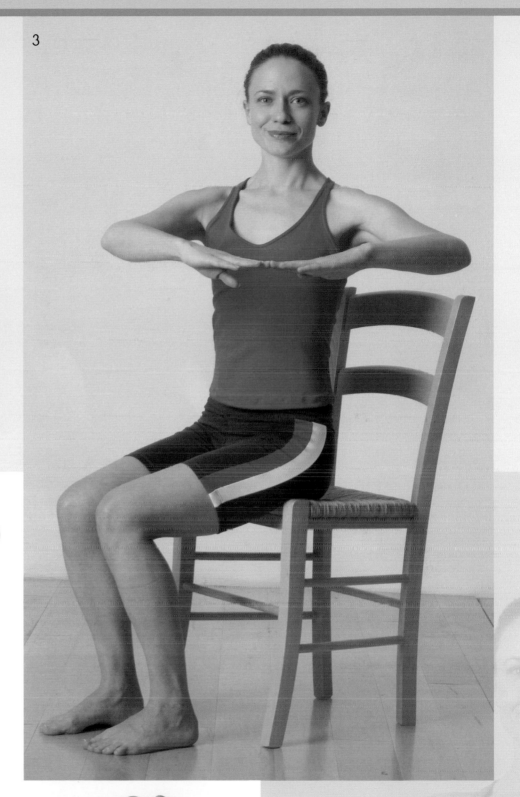

Challenge:

Spine Twist Knees Bent page 120.

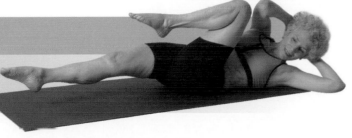

Hamstring Stretch Sitting

The Hamstring Stretch Sitting is a great warm-up stretch for the back of the thigh.

1 Sit at the front edge of the chair. Straighten your left leg and bend your right knee. You want the legs parallel to each other. Place both hands on the left leg, with your left foot flexed. Inhale to prepare.

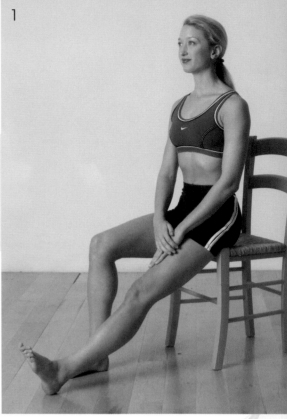

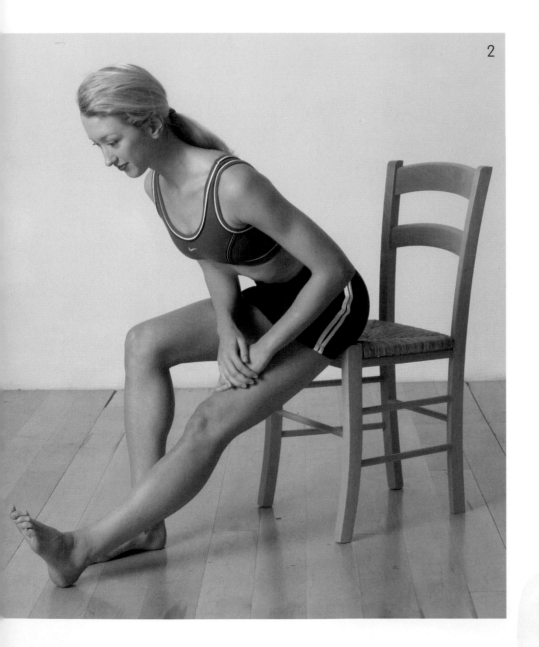

2 As you exhale, keep a flat back as you lengthen your upper torso towards your left leg. Inhale, keeping the back as flat as possible while lengthening through the top of the head.

3 As you exhale, slide your hands down the left leg. Reach towards the foot and think of placing the head on the knee.

4 Inhale up to a tall, flat back.

5 Repeat three times.

6 Repeat on the other side.

3

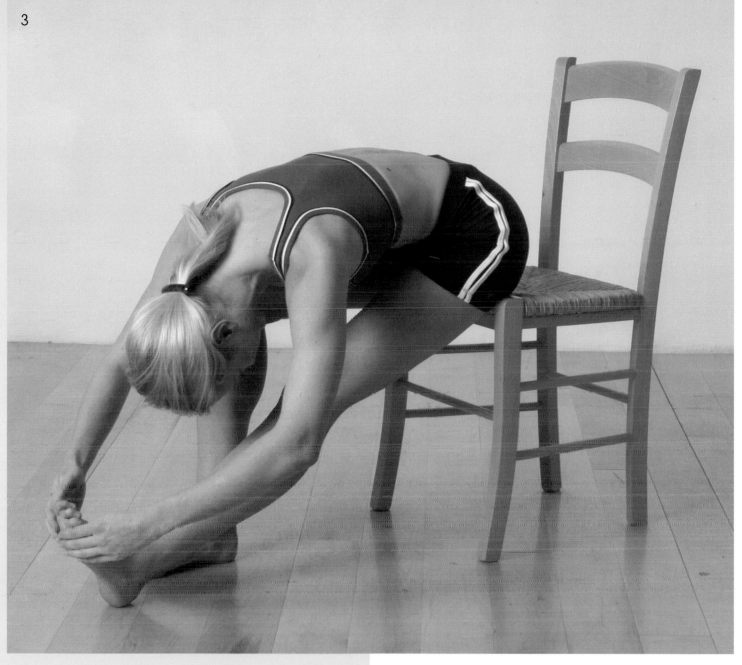

Key Points:

- Do not let your knee bend as you reach to the foot.

- Keep the shoulder blades pulling down the back.

- Keep the hips square as you lengthen forwards.

Challenge:

Hamstring Stretch
page 94.

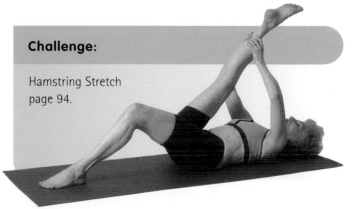

Pelvic Curl

The Pelvic Curl increases mobility of the spine and works on the connection between breath and movement.

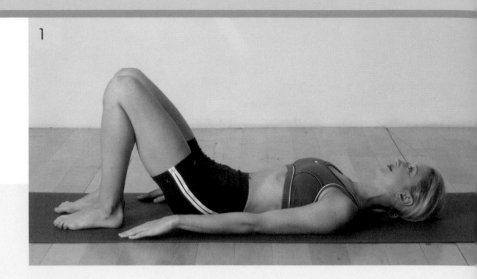

1 Start lying down on your back with your knees bent and your feet hip-width apart. Relax your arms down by your sides. Inhale to prepare.

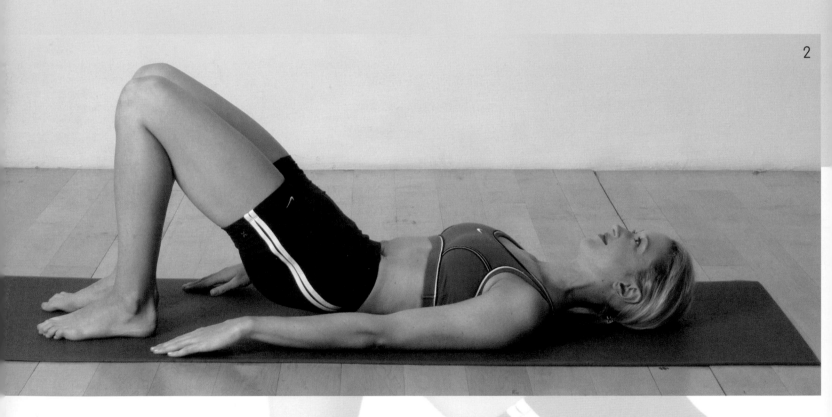

2 As you exhale, pull your navel into your spine and roll your tailbone up off the mat, one vertebra at a time.

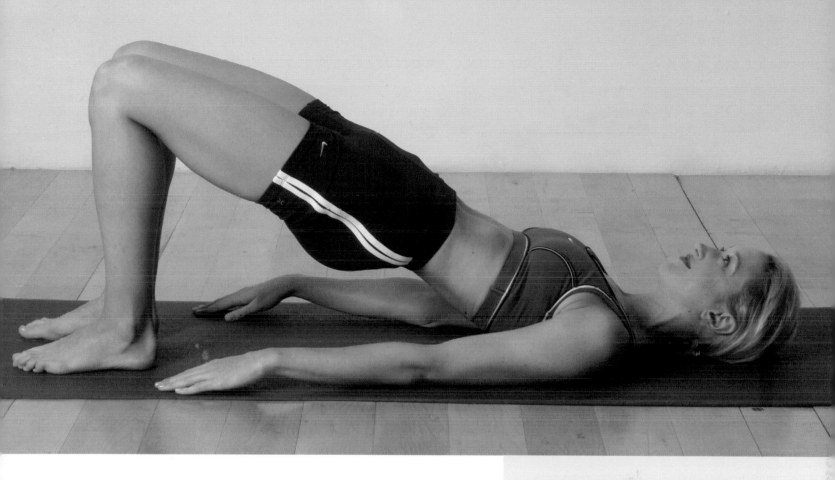

3 Keep the pelvis high while maintaining this bridge position as you inhale.

4 When you are ready to exhale, start rolling back down to the mat trying to feel each vertebra relax into the mat one at a time.

5 Inhale when the pelvis is back down on the ground.

6 Repeat five times.

Key Points:

- Make sure the neck is long and the chin is not crunched.
- Keep the knees parallel and hip-width apart.
- Do not roll in or out on the feet.

Challenge:

Pelvic Curls with Arms, page 80.

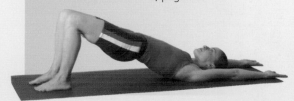

Abdominals

This exercise focuses on isolating the stomach while maintaining correct alignment. It is important to focus on pulling the abdominals in while curling forwards. This way, you get into the deep stomach muscles that support the spine. When the abdominal exercises are done correctly, they help alleviate lower back pain. By strengthening the deep muscles that support the spine, pressure is taken off the back.

1 Lie on your back with your knees bent and your feet flat on the floor. Your feet, knees, and hips should all be hip-width apart and parallel to each other.

2 Lace the fingers behind your head. Lift your elbows 5cm/2in. off the ground. Think of your arms as a hammock into which the head is relaxing. Inhale to prepare.

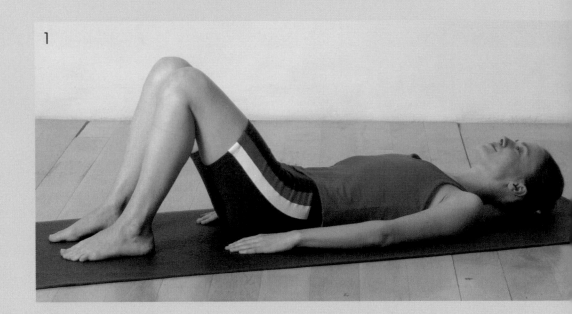

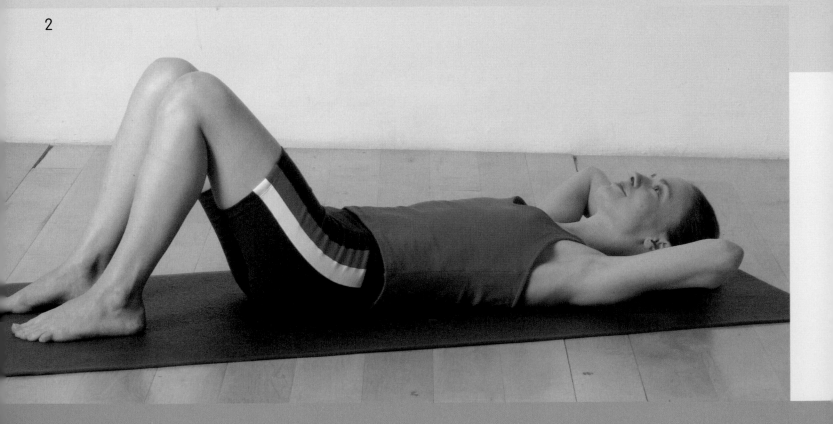

3 As you exhale, pull the navel down into the spine and lift the head up. Think of using the arms to lift the head, and keeping the pelvis still.

4 Inhale to relax down.

5 Repeat ten times.

Key Points:

- Relax the head back and use the back of your arms, or triceps, to lift the head; not your neck.

- Pull the shoulder blades down the back.

- Keep the feet and knees hip-width apart.

- Keep the navel pulling into the spine and breathe through the sides and back of the ribs.

- Do not let the pelvis tuck under as you curl forwards.

Challenge:

Intermediate Abdominals, page 82.

3

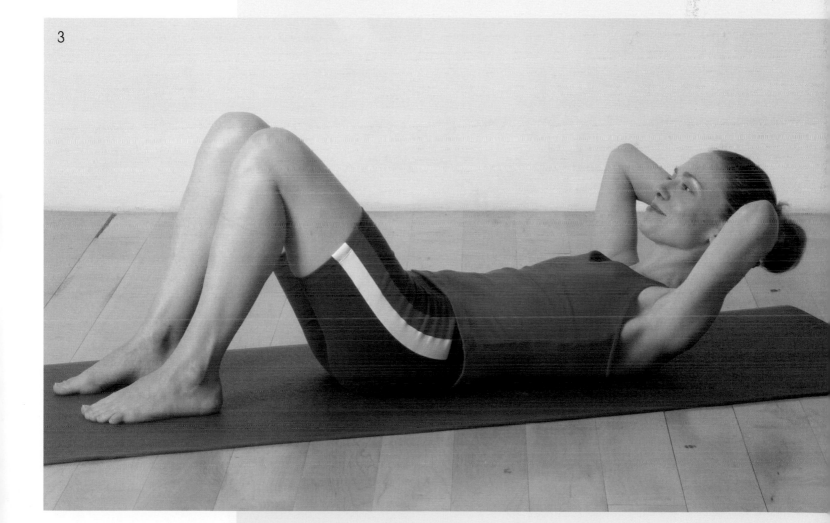

Obliques

This exercise flexes and rotates the torso as well as supporting the internal organs. Continue focusing on pulling in the abdominals as you exhale on the effort of the movement.

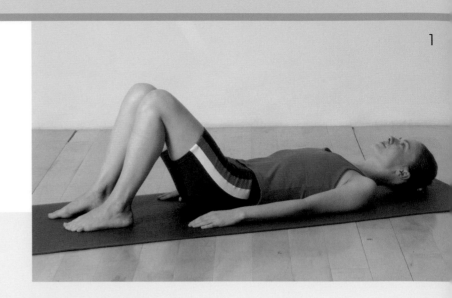

1 Lie on your back with your knees bent and your feet hip-width apart and parallel to each other.

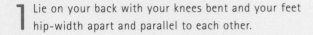

2 Lace your fingers behind your head and lift your elbows 5cm/2in. off the mat. Relax your head back in your hands and try not to use your neck muscles. Inhale to prepare.

3 As you exhale, curl forwards on the diagonal aiming for your left knee. Ideally you want to think of both shoulders coming off the mat.

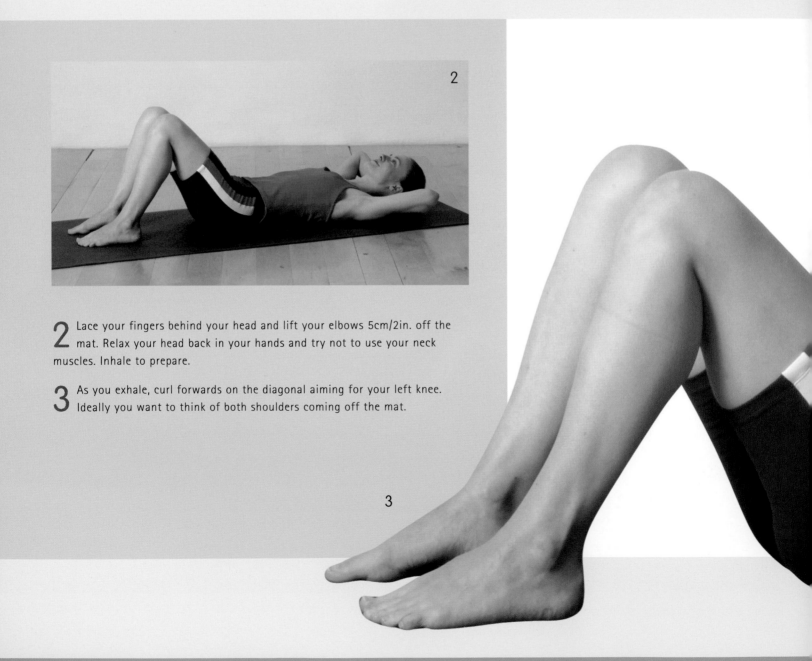

4 Inhale to relax down.

5 As you take your next exhale, twist up on the opposite diagonal and aim your elbows for your right knee.

6 Inhale to relax back down.

7 Repeat the right and left sides ten times.

Key Points:

- Try not to rest on your shoulders! Think of both shoulder blades pulling down the back as you twist.

- Relax the head back in your hands.

- Keep the feet and knees hip-width apart.

- Do not let the pelvis tilt as you round the upper torso forwards.

Challenge:

Advanced Abdominals with Twist, page 84

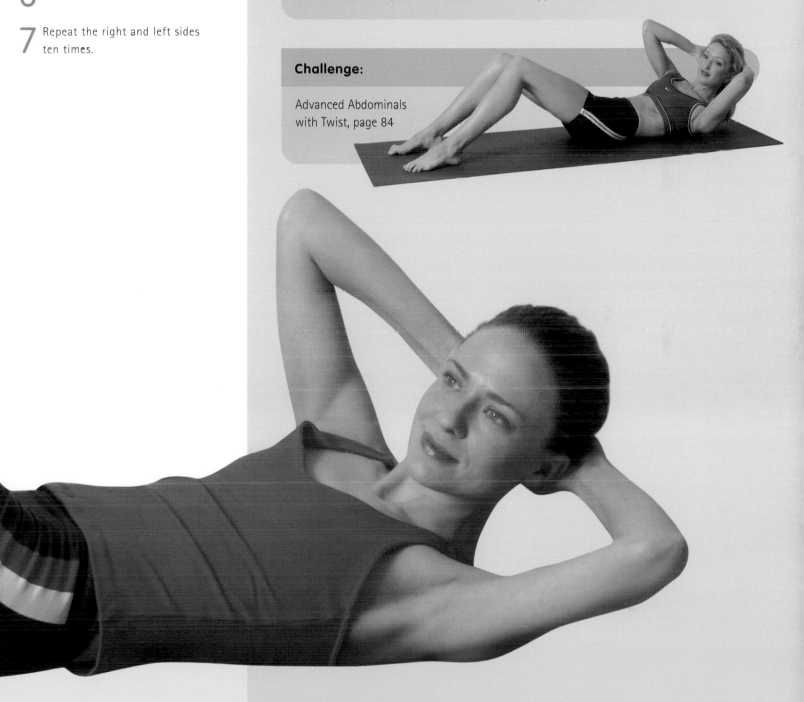

Buttocks Squeeze

The Buttocks Squeeze focuses on the connection between your abdominals and your sit bones as well as isolating your buttocks and hamstring muscles. You may find it more comfortable to place a small flat pillow under your hips.

1 Lie on your stomach. Rest your forehead on your hands and relax your shoulders. Keep your legs straight and parallel. Take a breath, inhaling.

2 As you exhale, pull your navel into your spine while squeezing your sit bones together. Your back will naturally relax and elongate.

3 As you inhale, relax everything back to a neutral position.

4 Repeat ten times.

Key Points:

- Make sure you are not holding tension in your shoulders.

- Keep the back relaxed at all times.

- Keep the legs parallel as you squeeze the buttocks.

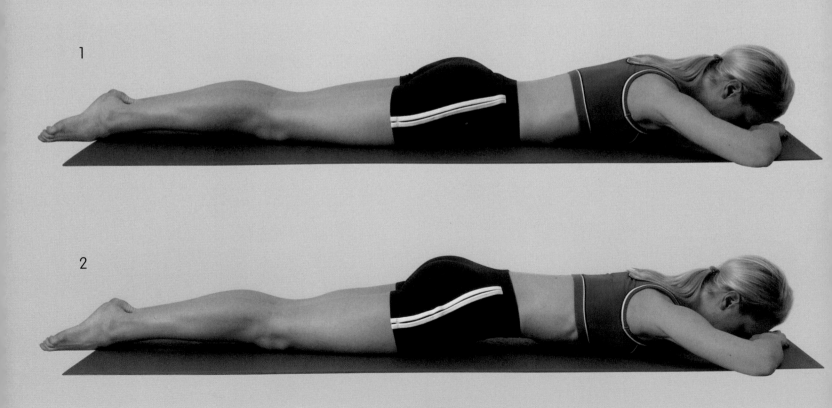

Shoulder Blades

The Shoulder Blades exercise is designed to isolate the muscles of the back: rhomboids, trapezius, and latissimus dorsi.

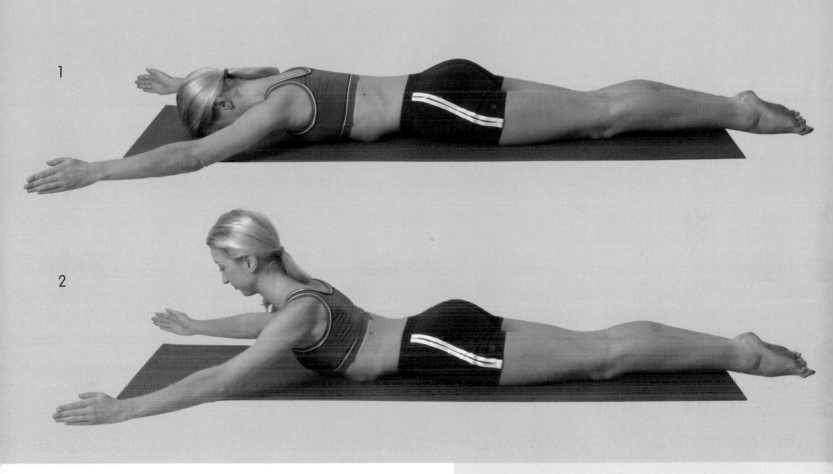

1 Lie on your stomach with your legs out straight and squeezed tight together. Place your arms in a high diagonal on the ground so that they form a V position – palms facing each other. Inhale to prepare.

2 As you exhale, pull the navel into your spine and your shoulder blades back and down. Slightly lift your head and upper torso. Your arms should stay straight.

3 Inhale to relax the shoulders, neck and head.

4 Repeat five times.

Key Points:

- Keep the navel pulling into the spine and breathe through the sides and back of the ribs.

- Keep your neck long.

- Keep your arms straight.

- Do not arch your lower back.

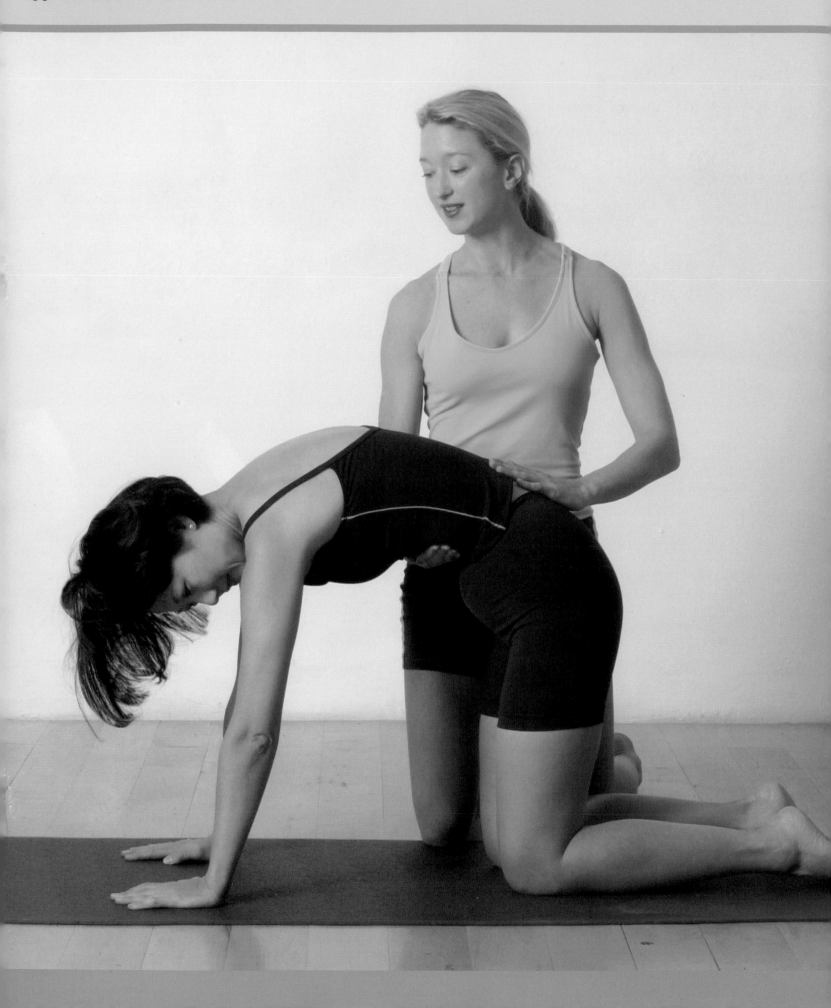

Cat

The Cat focuses on increasing mobility of the spine.

1 Place your hands and knees on the floor with your hands directly underneath your shoulders and your knees hip-width apart. Inhale to prepare.

2 As you exhale, round your back towards the ceiling and relax your head forwards. As you inhale, relax your back into neutral.

3 As you exhale, arch your back and look straight ahead keeping your abdominals in.

4 As you inhale, relax back to neutral.

5 Repeat this exercise five times.

Key Points:

- If you have back problems, leave out the arch. Just do the first two points of the exercise.

- Keep the shoulder blades down the back as you exhale

- Make sure your hands and knees stay shoulder- and hip-width apart.

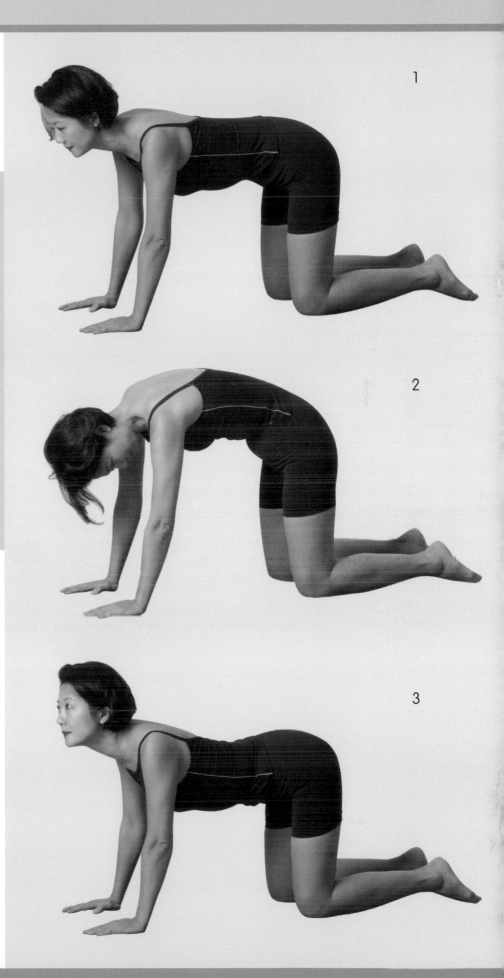

1

2

3

Child's Pose

The Child's Pose is a wonderful stretch for your back and upper torso.

1 Bend your knees and sit on your heels. Stretch your arms out in front of you and relax your upper torso forwards so that your upper body is resting on your lower. Take three deep breaths.

Key Points:

- If you have problems with your knees please leave this exercise out.

- Let your natural body weight stretch out the spine.

- Keep the shoulders relaxed.

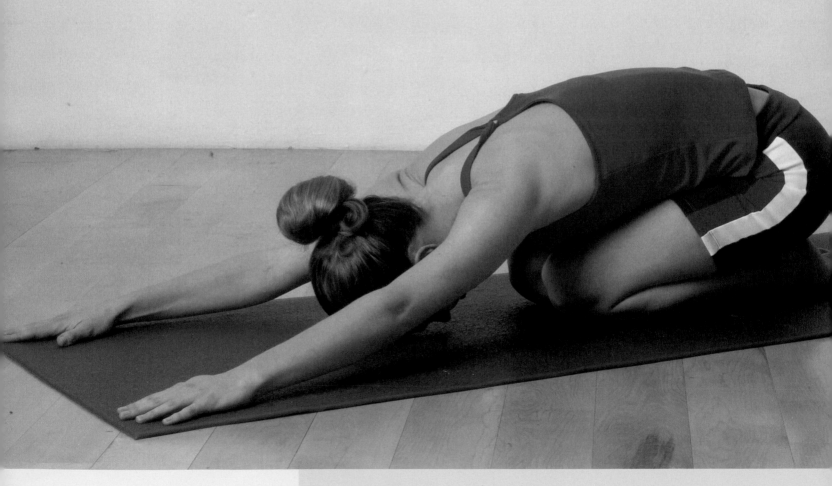

Abdominal Isolation

Abdominal Isolation is a great exercise for learning to work from the powerhouse when moving the limbs. The purpose of this exercise is to focus on the movement of the legs initiating from the abdominals. Work on finding the connection between the leg and the stomach muscles, and it will form one of the building blocks for the more challenging exercises! You may find it more comfortable to rest your head on a pillow.

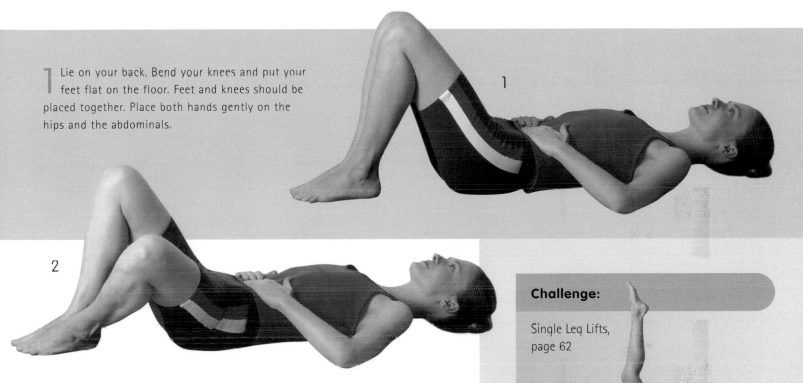

1 Lie on your back. Bend your knees and put your feet flat on the floor. Feet and knees should be placed together. Place both hands gently on the hips and the abdominals.

2 As you inhale, open your left knee to the side, making sure the back and hip do not move. You are opening the knee as much as possible, while keeping the rest of the body still. As you exhale, pull the navel into the spine to bring the knee back up to the centre.

3 Immediately repeat to the right side.

4 Alternate sides, repeating the whole exercise eight times.

Key Points:

- Keep the shoulders down and the neck long.
- Lengthen the crown of the head away from the tailbone.

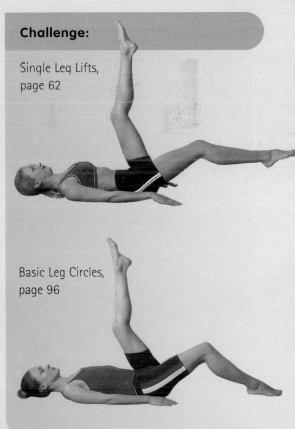

Challenge:

Single Leg Lifts, page 62

Basic Leg Circles, page 96

Abdominals with Arm Extension

The Abdominals with Arm Extension is a more challenging variation of the basic Abdominals exercise (see page 50). Not only do you have to think of the abdominals pulling in as you curl forwards, but the exercise works on isolating the biceps and shoulder blades as well.

1 Lie on your back and bend your knees, feet hip-width apart and parallel to each other. Lace your fingers behind your head. Lift your elbows 5cm/2in. off the mat and relax your head back in your hands. Take a deep breath, inhaling.

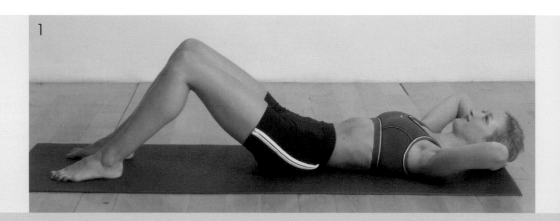

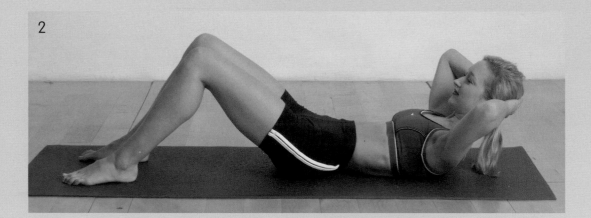

2 As you exhale pull your navel into your spine and lift your head and shoulders up with your arms.

3 Stay where you are. As you inhale, extend your arms to hold on to the backs of your thighs.

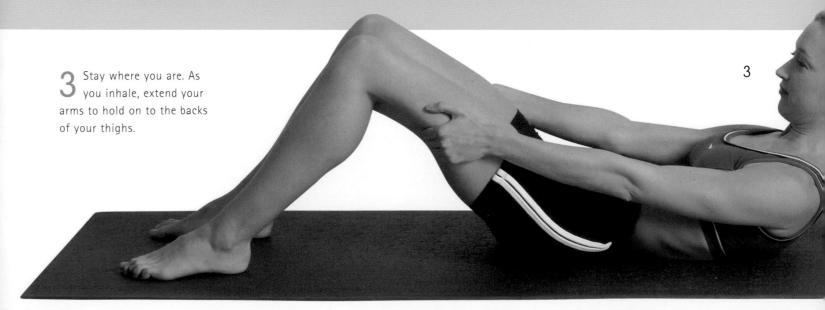

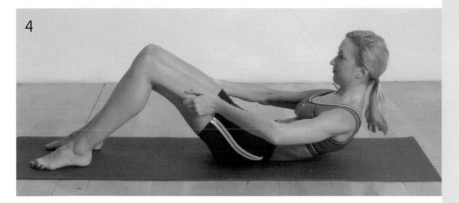

4 As you exhale, bend your elbows out to the side and scoop the abdominals down towards your spine. You should feel your arms really working.

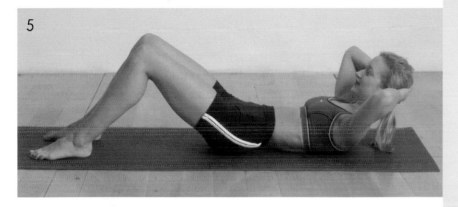

5 Stay where you are. As you inhale, bring the hands back behind the head without dropping.

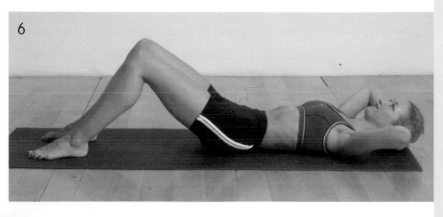

6 Exhale and stay where you are, trying to recreate the scoop you had with your hands behind your legs. Inhale to relax.

7 Repeat five times.

Key Points:

- Curl up high enough so that there is no pressure on the back of the neck.

- Keep the navel pulling into the spine and breathe through the sides and back of the ribs.

- Keep the shoulder blades pulling down the back.

- Keep the feet and knees hip-width apart.

- Do not let the upper torso drop during the exercise.

- Do not let the pelvis tuck under as you round forwards.

Progression from:

Abdominals, page 50.

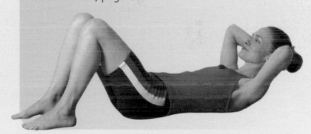

Challenge:

Elementary Single Leg Stretch, page 100.

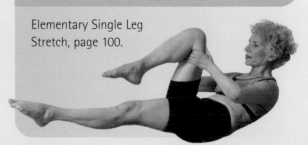

Single Leg Lifts

The Single Leg Lifts exercise is a more difficult variation of the Abdominal Isolation (see page 50). Although both exercises focus on controlling the legs from the abdominal muscles, Single Leg Lifts requires more flexibility in the hip and stabilization of the spine.

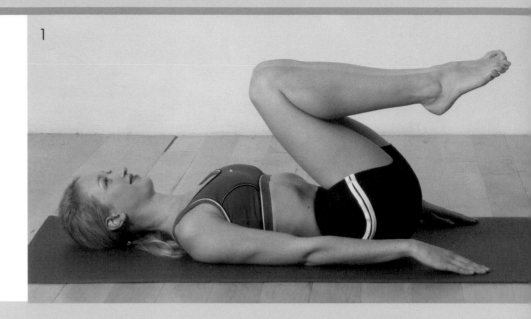

1

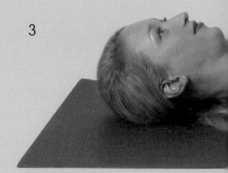

2

3

1 Lie on your back with your knees bent into your chest and your arms down by your sides.

2 Inhale and stretch your legs towards the ceiling, keeping the knees slightly bent.

3 As you exhale, pull the navel into the spine and slowly bring the right leg down towards the floor. Lower the leg to a 45 degree angle to the floor.

4 Inhale and bring the leg back up towards the ceiling.

5 On your second exhale, lower the left leg down towards the floor.

6 Repeat five times each leg.

Key Points:

- Make sure the back stays flat into the floor at all times.
- Keep the shoulder blades pulling down the back.
- Keep the neck long.
- Keep the navel pulling into the spine and breathe through the sides and back of the ribs.

Progression from:

Abdominal Isolation, page 59.

Challenge:

Double Bent Leg Stretch, page 104.

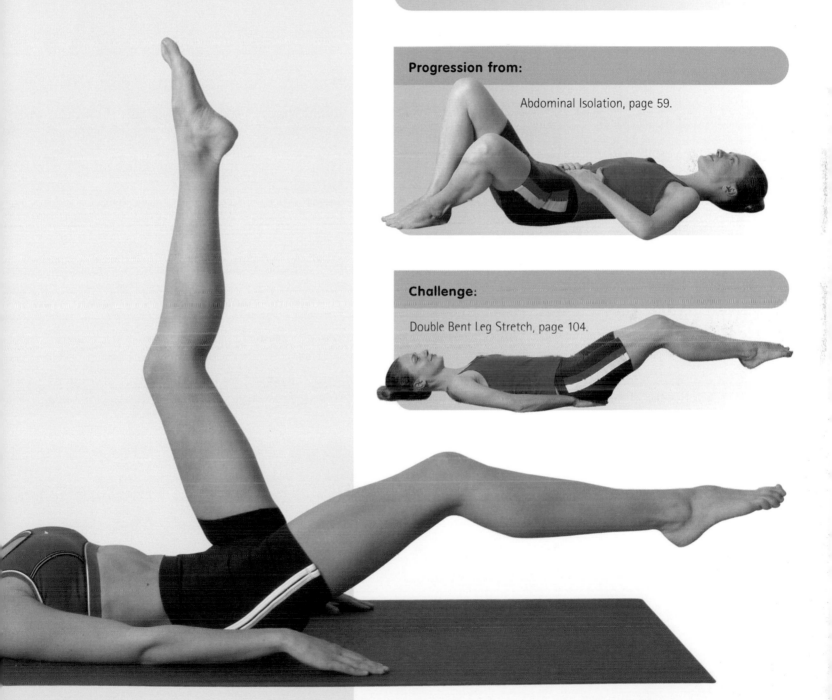

Pelvic Curls with Leg Lifts

This exercise requires stability in the powerhouse. It isolates the hamstrings while focusing on the deep stabilization of the abdominal muscles.

1 Lie on your back with your knees bent and feet hip-width apart. Lengthen your arms down by your sides. Inhale to prepare.

2 As you exhale, slowly roll the pelvis off the ground into the bridge position. Keep the pressure on your feet equal and do not roll them in and out.

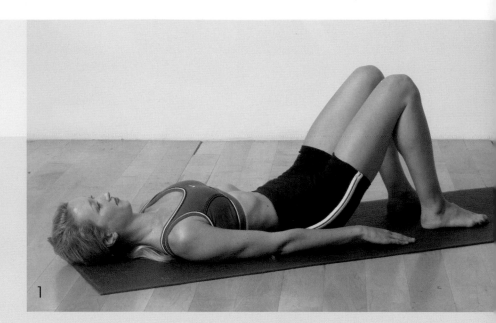

1

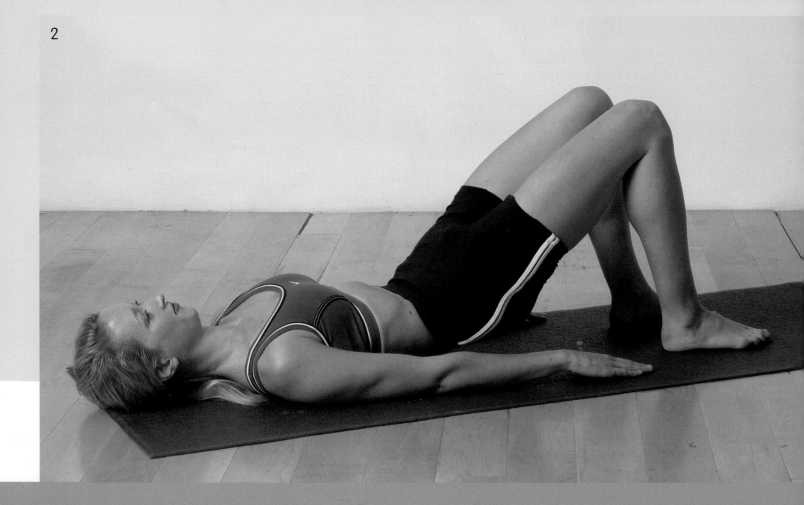

2

3

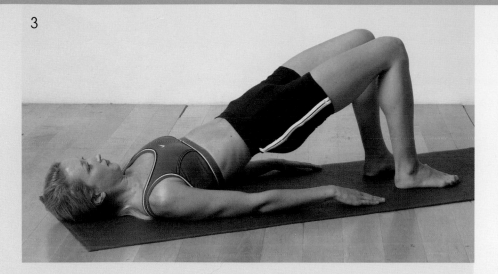

3 Inhale, staying in this position. The most important part of the exercise is to keep the hips square. Do not let one hip drop lower than the other.

4 As you exhale, lift the right foot up off the ground 5cm/2in.

5 Inhale to relax the foot back to the mat keeping the hips still.

6 As you exhale, lift the left foot off the ground 5cm/2in. You should be feeling the hamstrings on the right side working to keep the hips square.

7 Repeat three times on each side..

4

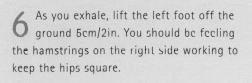

Key Points:

- Make sure the hips do not drop!

- Keep the buttocks squeezed.

- Keep the navel pulling into the spine and breathe through the sides and back of the ribs.

- Keep the shoulder blades pulling down the back, and your arms long.

Challenge:

Shoulder Bridge, page 194.

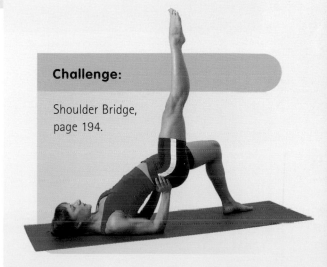

Inner Thigh

This exercise is designed to isolate and strengthen the inner thighs. Focus on the connection between your breath and the movement of the leg. You may find this more comfortable If you place a small pillow under your head, and one under your leg.

1 Lie on the floor. Place your left arm underneath your head. Bend the right leg so that the thigh is at a right angle to your torso. Extend your left leg straight so that your head, hips and bottom leg are all in a straight line. Place your right hand on your hip and make sure the hip stays stable. Inhale to prepare.

2 As you exhale, pull your navel into your spine and lift your bottom leg towards the ceiling. You should feel the abdominals and inner thigh engaging.

3 Inhale to relax completely.

4 Repeat the exercise five to ten times.

5 Repeat on the other side.

Key Points:

- Keep the hips square. Do not let the top hip roll forwards or backwards.

- Keep the shoulders relaxed and down.

- Keep the navel pulling into the spine and breathe through the sides and back of the ribs.

- Keep the back straight.

- Lengthen out through the top of the head.

- Extend through the toes.

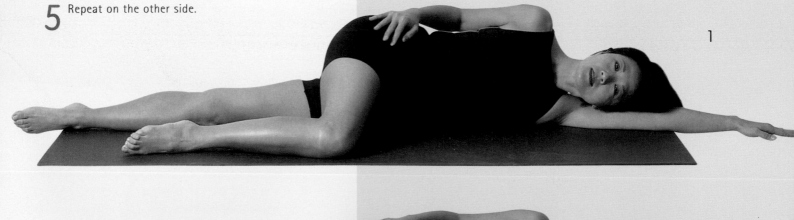

1

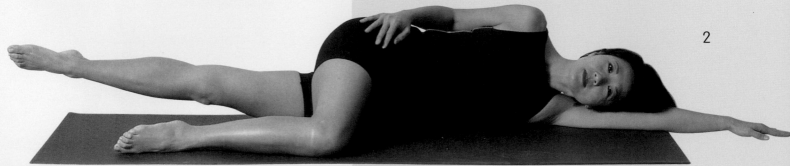

2

Triceps

This exercise is for strengthening the backs of the arms, the triceps.

You will need: two small weights. Women please use no more than 2kg/5lb weights, men 3kg/7lb. You may also find it more comfortable to place a small pillow under your head.

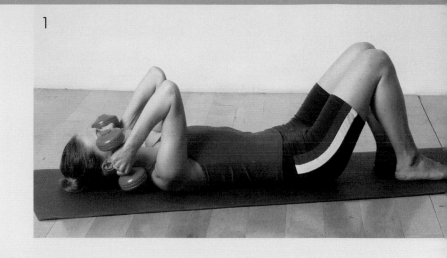

1

1 Lie on your back. Place the feet flat on the floor with your feet, knees and hips all in one line. Place one weight in each hand, and bend your arms so that the hands are by your ears and the elbows are parallel and pointed to the ceiling. Inhale to prepare.

2 As you exhale, make sure the elbows do not move in space and straighten your arms to the ceiling.

3 Inhale to relax your forearms back to the original position.

4 Repeat ten times.

Key Points:

- Keep the navel pulling into the spine and breathe through the sides and back of the ribs.
- Keep the shoulder blades pulling down.
- Keep the feet and knees hip-width apart.
- Do not tuck the pelvis.
- Make sure the elbows do not move in space.

Challenge:

Triceps Push-ups, page 122

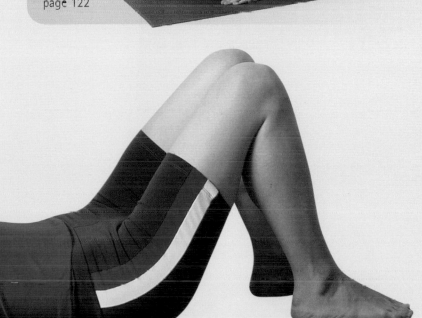

2

Karate Chops

This exercise is a slightly different variation of the triceps. Think about keeping the shoulders down while connecting the breath with the movement.

You will need: two small weights. Women please use no more than 2kg5?lb, men 3kg/7lb. You may also be more comfortable with a small pillow under your head.

1 Lie on your back. Bend your knees and place your feet flat on the floor. Make sure your feet, knees and hips are all in alignment. Place one weight in your right hand. Place your right hand on your left shoulder. The elbow and shoulder should be in alignment with the elbow facing the ceiling. Place the left hand below the right elbow for stabilization. Drop your shoulders down your back. Inhale to prepare.

2 As you exhale, pull the navel into the spine and extend your right hand towards the ceiling. Make sure the right elbow does not move in space.

3 Inhale and relax the right arm back to the nape of the neck on the left side.

4 Repeat ten times.

5 Repeat on the other side.

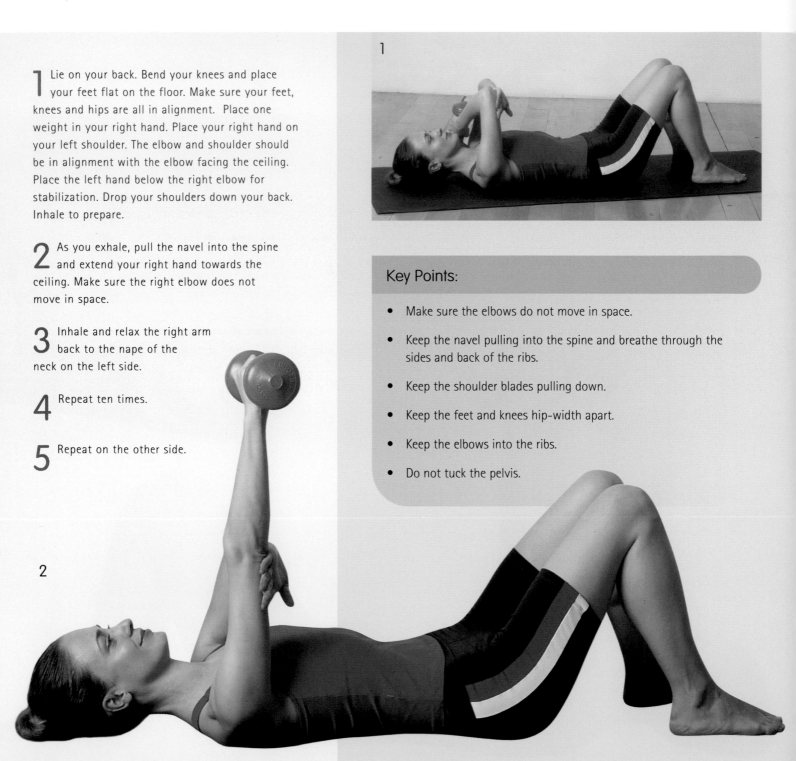

1

2

Key Points:

- Make sure the elbows do not move in space.

- Keep the navel pulling into the spine and breathe through the sides and back of the ribs.

- Keep the shoulder blades pulling down.

- Keep the feet and knees hip-width apart.

- Keep the elbows into the ribs.

- Do not tuck the pelvis.

Teaser with Feet on the Chair

The Teaser with Feet on the Chair begins to put all the isolations of various muscle groups together. Focus on working the whole body in one graceful movement. The inner thighs are squeezing, the abdominals are pulling in, and the shoulder blades are pulling down the back on the exhale.

You will need: one small pillow.

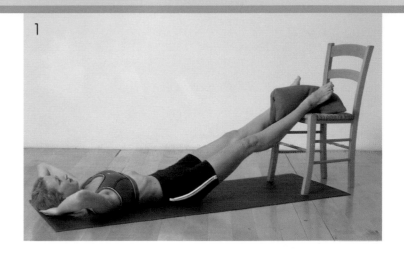

1 Lie on your back with your feet on a chair at a 45-degree angle and your legs straight. Place a pillow between your feet, with your toes on the outside and your heels on the inside. Lace the fingers behind your head and lift your elbows slightly off the mat. Take a breath, inhaling.

2 As you exhale, simultaneously pull your navel into your spine, squeeze the pillow with your heels and slowly curl the upper torso forwards.

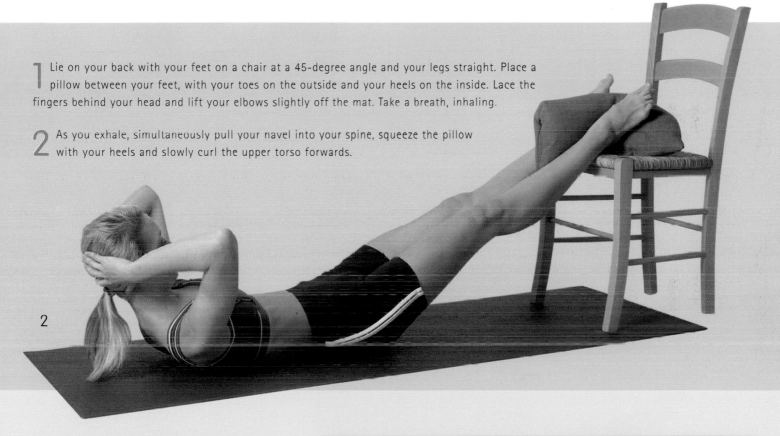

3 As you inhale, relax everything back to the starting position.

4 Repeat ten times.

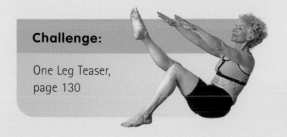

Challenge:

One Leg Teaser, page 130

Key Points:

- Try to think of everything working together.
- Keep the navel pulling into the spine and breathe through the sides and back of the ribs.
- Keep the hips neutral. Do not tuck the hips as you curl forwards.
- Keep the shoulder blades pulling down the back.
- Squeeze the buttocks and inner thighs together.

Hip Stretch 1

This is a great stretch for the hip, especially the piriformis, the muscle that does most of the work when turning out the leg. When problems arise it can cause sciatica – shooting pains down the back of the leg.

1 Lie on your back with your feet planted on the floor and your knees bent. Cross your right ankle across your left knee. Take both hands and hold on to the underside of your left thigh.

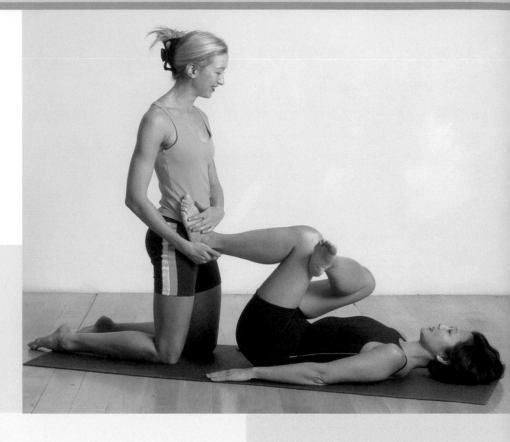

2 Pull the left thigh into your chest. Take three deep breaths.

3 Change to the other side.

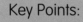

Key Points:

- Keep the navel pulling into the spine and breathe through the sides and back of the ribs.

- Keep the pelvis flat as you pull the knee towards the chest.

- Keep the shoulder blades pulling down the back.

Hip Stretch 2

This exercise is a nice stretch to release the outside of your hip.

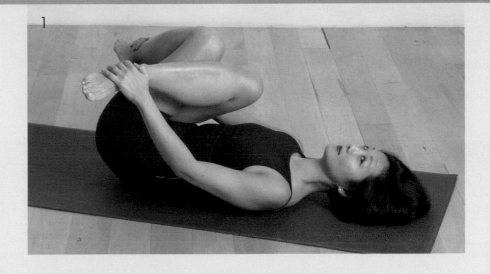

1 Lie on your back and cross the right knee over the left. Bring your knees straight into your chest. Hold on to your right ankle with your left hand and your left ankle with your right hand. Inhale to prepare.

2 As you exhale, pull your feet towards your shoulders. You should feel a stretch in your right hip.

3 Repeat three times.

4 Repeat on the other side.

Key Points:

- If you have knee problems, leave this exercise out.

- Keep the navel pulling into the spine and breathe through the sides and back of the ribs.

- Keep the pelvis flat as you pull the knee towards the chest.

- Keep the shoulder blades pulling down the back.

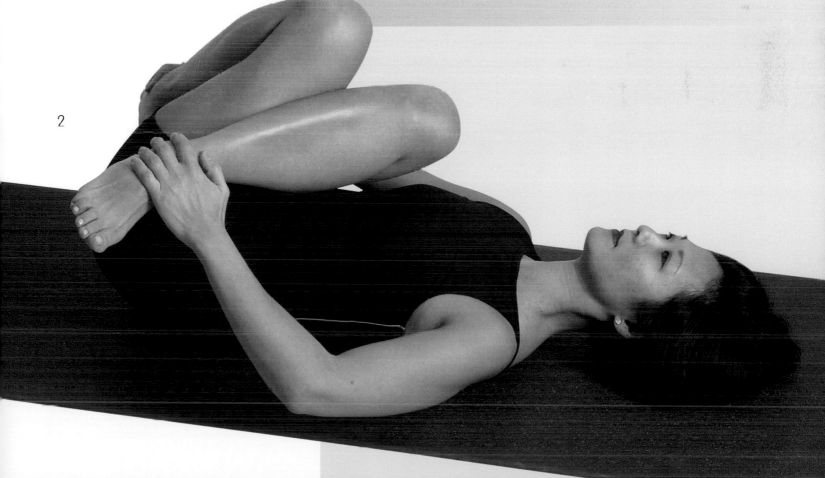

Beginner's 15-minute workout

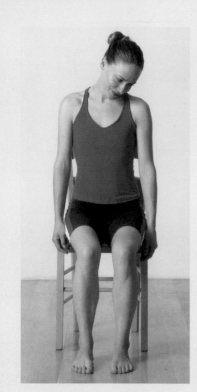

Head Circles page 36

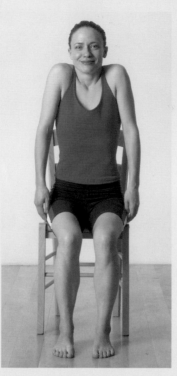

Shoulder Shrugs page 38

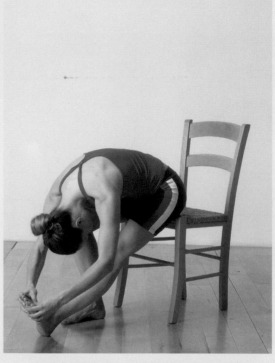

Hamstring Stretch Sitting page 46

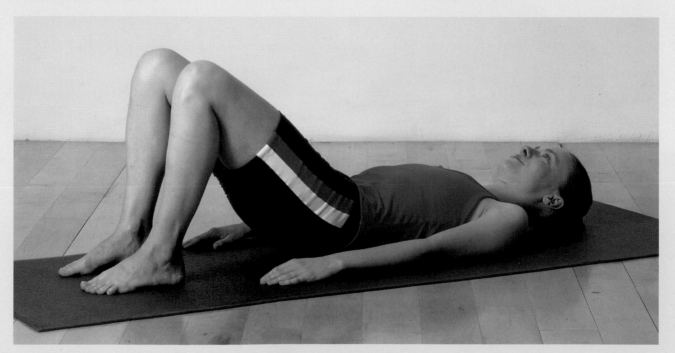

Pelvic curl page 48

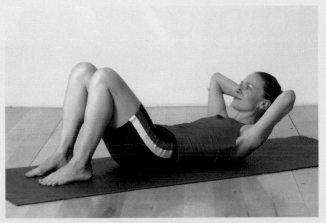

Abdominals page 50

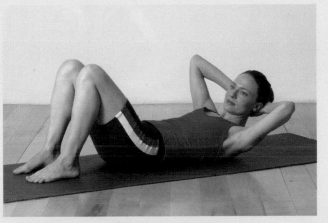

Obliques page 52

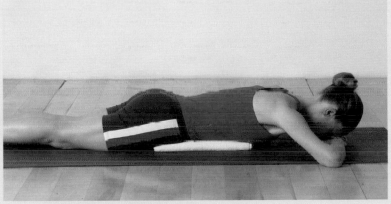

Buttocks Squeeze page 54

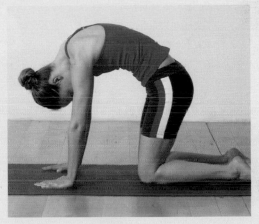

Cat page 56

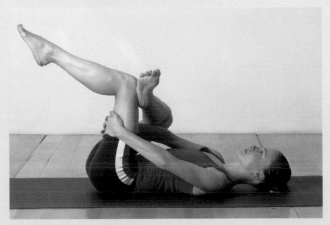

Hip Stretch 1 page 70

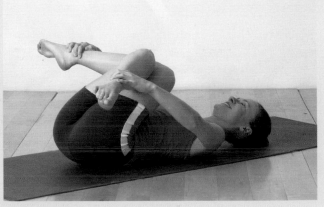

Hip Stretch 2 page 71

Intermediate

'True flexibility can be achieved only when all muscles are uniformly developed.'

Joseph Pilates

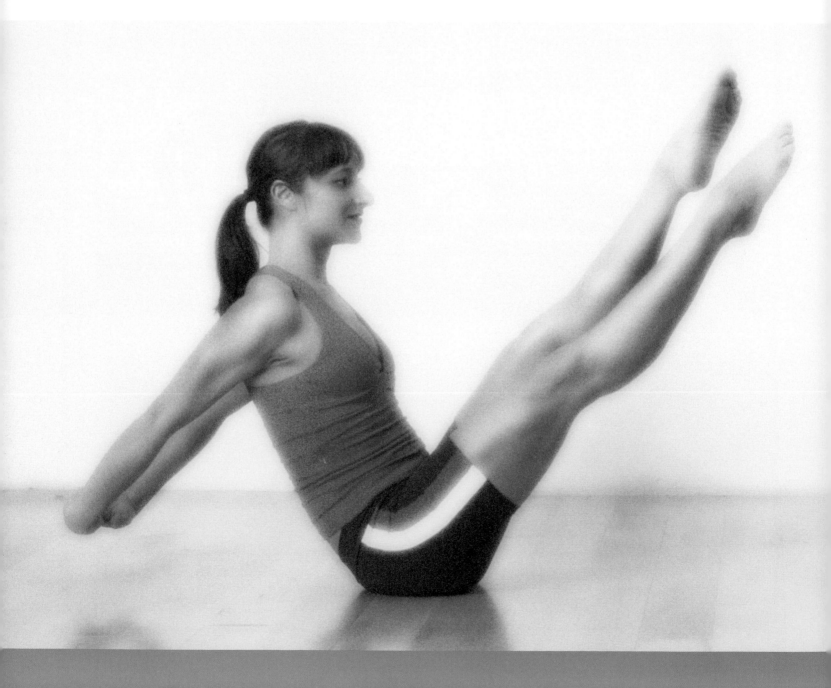

'Pilates is the single best way I know to slow down the ageing process, no matter what age you begin. In the four years I have been doing Pilates, and I am now 62, in addition to increased flexibility and strength, I have lost inches off my waist, thighs, legs and hips, have firmed my stomach and stretched and lengthened my calves. And best of all, no matter how sad or gloomy I might feel when I begin, the very act of doing the exercises raises my spirits and leaves me with a new vigour and cheerful attitude.'

Linda Daitz

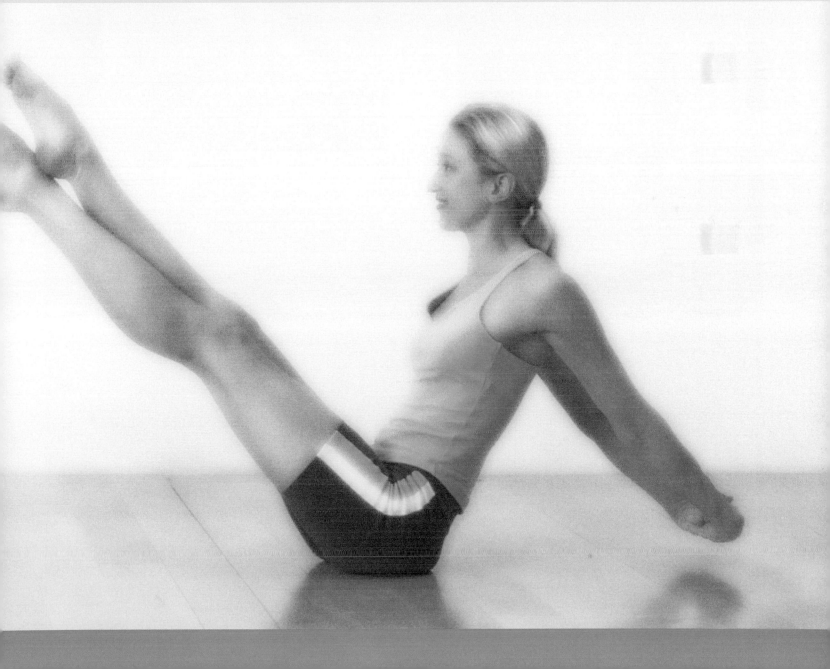

Introduction

The intermediate section is a combination of the various Pilates exercises taught internationally. This section develops from the previous section by starting to integrate all the isolations into a fluid, continuous whole. The exercises that were originally taught by Joseph Pilates are clearly marked with the symbol (*). If the exercise is an adaptation of an original exercise, you will find the same symbol together with a note at the bottom of the page. This means that the exercise is taught in a studio which uses the original method, but has been modified.

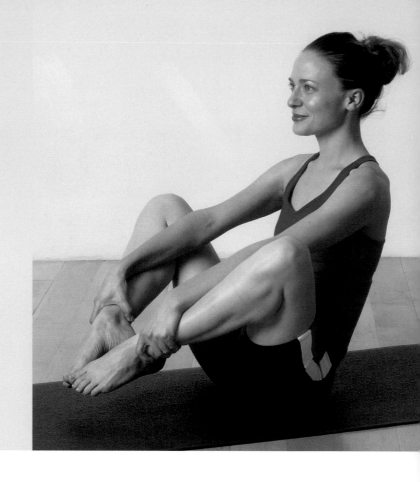

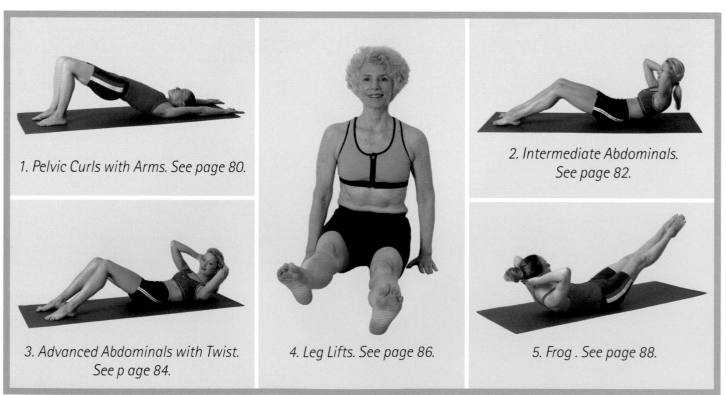

1. Pelvic Curls with Arms. See page 80.

2. Intermediate Abdominals. See page 82.

3. Advanced Abdominals with Twist. See p age 84.

4. Leg Lifts. See page 86.

5. Frog . See page 88.

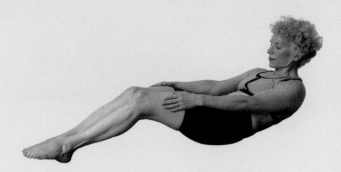

6. Elementary Hundred. See page 90.

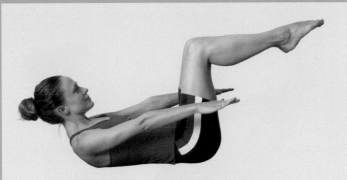

7. Basic Roll-up . See page 92.

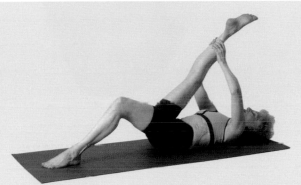

8. Hamstring Stretch. See page 94.

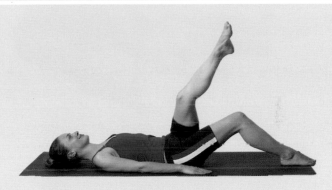

9. Basic Leg Circles. See page 96.

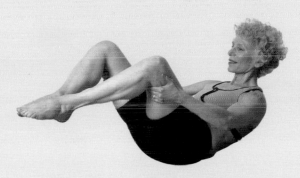

10. Rolling Like a Ball Open. See page 98.

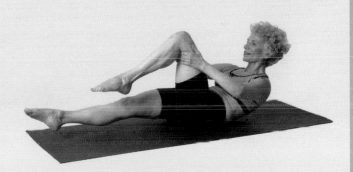

11. Elementary Single Leg Stretch. See page 100.

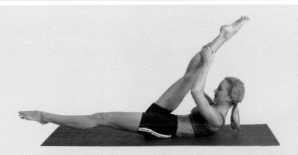

12. Single Straight Leg Stretch. See page 103.

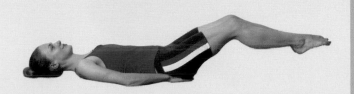

13. Double Bent Leg Stretch. See page 104.

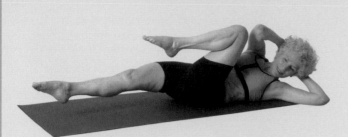

14. Criss Cross. See page 106.

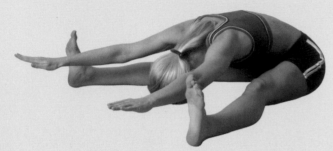

15. Spine Stretch Forward. See page 108.

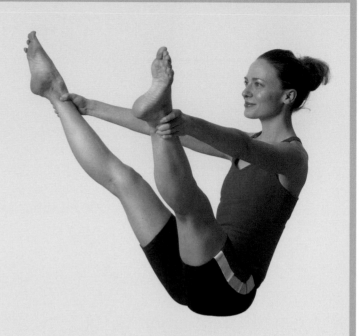

16. Prep for Open Leg Rocker. See page 110.

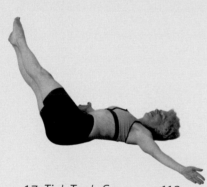

17. Tick Tock. See page 112.

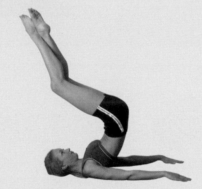

18. Pelvic Lifts Ankles Crossed.
See page 114.

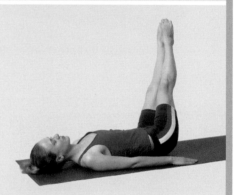

19. Small Corkscrew. See page 116.

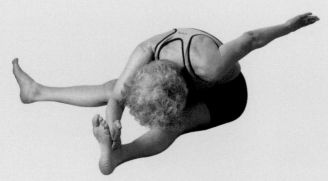

20. Saw. See page 118.

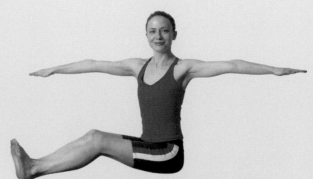

21. Spine Twist Knees Bent. See page 120.

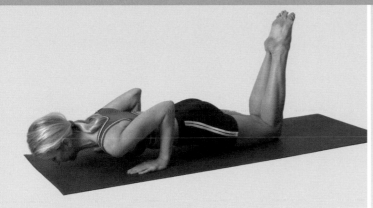

22. Triceps Push-ups. See page 122.

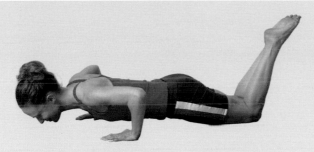

23. Shoulder and Pecs Push-ups See page 124.

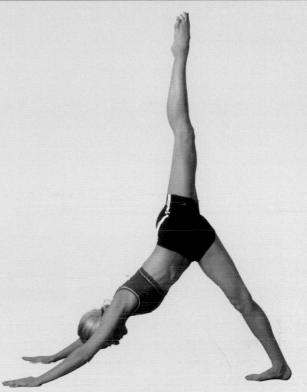

24. Arabesque. See page 126.

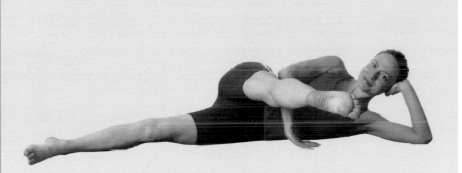

25. Side Kicks. See page 128.

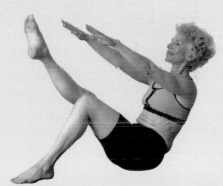

26. One Leg Teaser. See page 130.

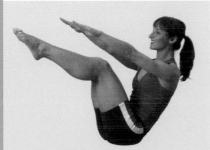

27. Teaser Knees Bent.
    See page 132.

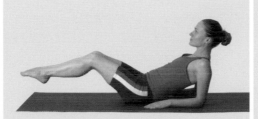

28. Teaser 2 on Elbows. See page 134.

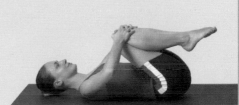

29. Hug Knees to Chest. See page 138.

Pelvic Curls with Arms

This exercise is the next development of the basic Pelvic Curls. Focus on releasing the back while lengthening the spine and stretching the shoulders.

1 Lie on your back with your knees bent and your feet hip-width apart. Place your arms down by your sides. Take a breath, inhaling.

2 As you exhale, pull the navel into the spine and slowly roll the tailbone off the mat.

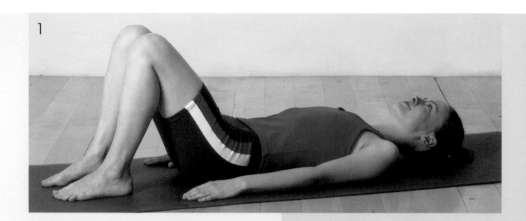

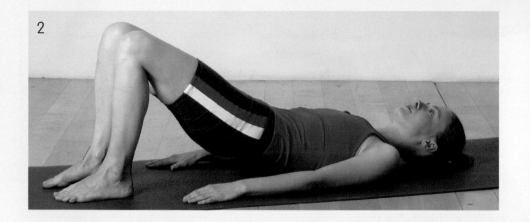

3 Keeping the pelvis high as you inhale, raise your arms lengthening through your hands over your head to the ground behind you. Only reach your hands as far back as is comfortable.

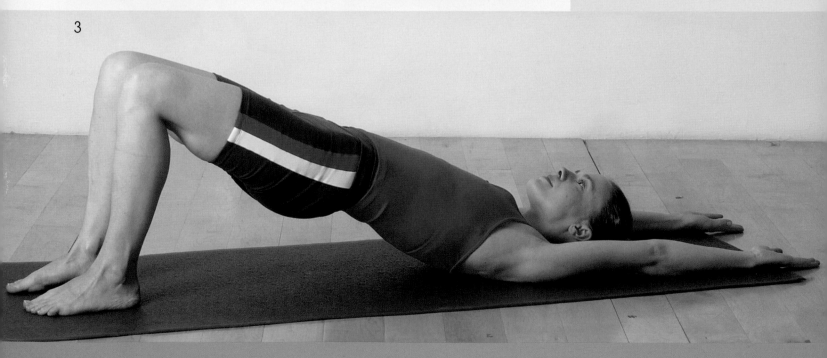

4 Keeping your hands reaching over your head, exhale and roll the pelvis back down the mat one vertebra at a time.

5 Keep the pelvis flat on the ground as you inhale and lower the arms sideways and down to the hips. Make sure you are moving the arms from the back and not arching your back or letting go of your ribs.

4

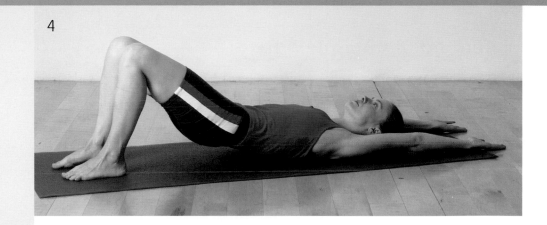

5

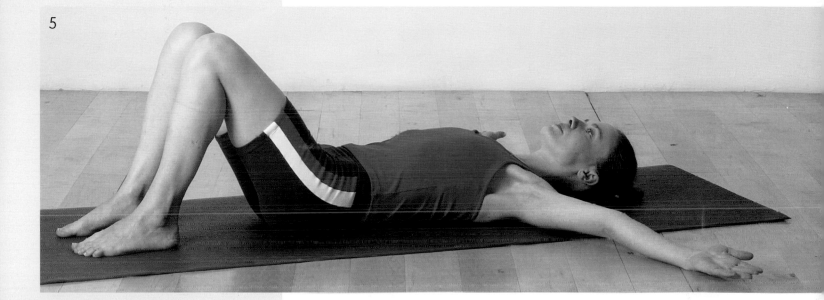

Key Points:

- Make sure the back rounds up and down one vertebra at a time.

- Keep the knees and feet hip-width apart.

- Keep the navel pulling into your spine and breathe through the sides and back of the ribs.

- Extend through your fingertips.

- Do not arch the ribs as you pull the shoulder blades and arms down by your sides.

- Do not roll in or out on your feet.

6 Repeat five times.

Progression from: Beginner's Pelvic Curl, page 48

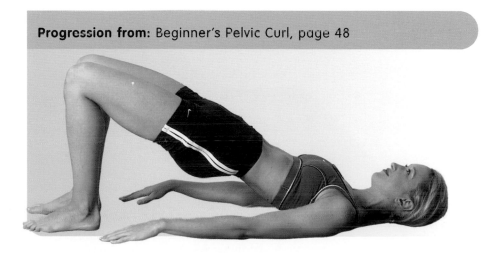

Intermediate Abdominals

The Intermediate Abdominals are a more difficult variation of the basic Abdominals. Continue focusing on lengthening and pulling the stomach down, while curling the upper torso forwards.

1 Lie on your back with your knees bent and your feet hip-width apart. Make sure your feet and knees are hip-width apart and parallel to each other. Lace the fingers behind the head with the elbows out to the sides. Take a breath, inhaling.

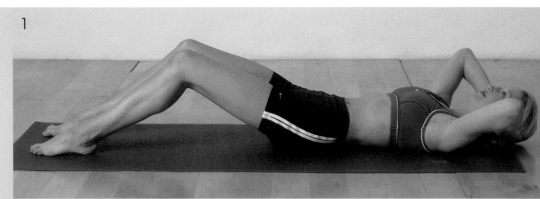

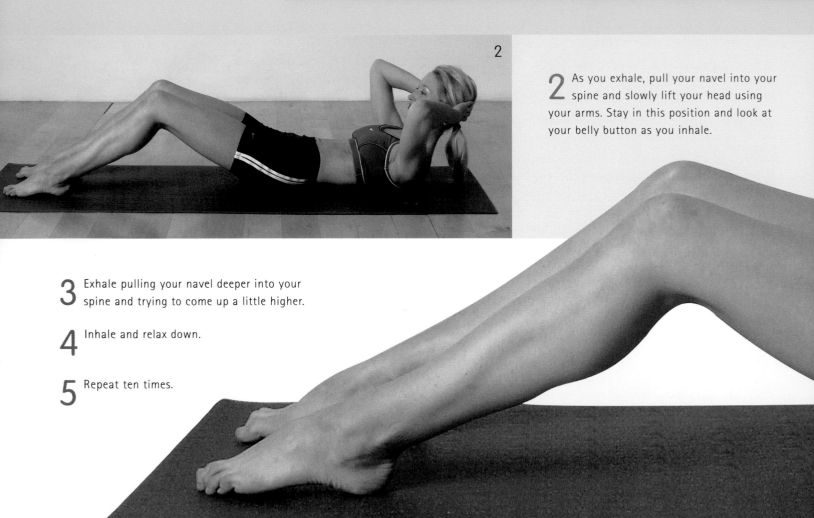

2 As you exhale, pull your navel into your spine and slowly lift your head using your arms. Stay in this position and look at your belly button as you inhale.

3 Exhale pulling your navel deeper into your spine and trying to come up a little higher.

4 Inhale and relax down.

5 Repeat ten times.

Key Points:

- Relax the head back in the hands.
- Pull the shoulder blades down the back.
- Keep the feet and knees hip-width apart.
- Keep the navel pulling into your spine and breathe through the sides and back of the ribs.
- Do not tense the neck!
- Do not tuck the pelvis as you curl forwards.

Progression from: Beginner's Abdominals, page 50

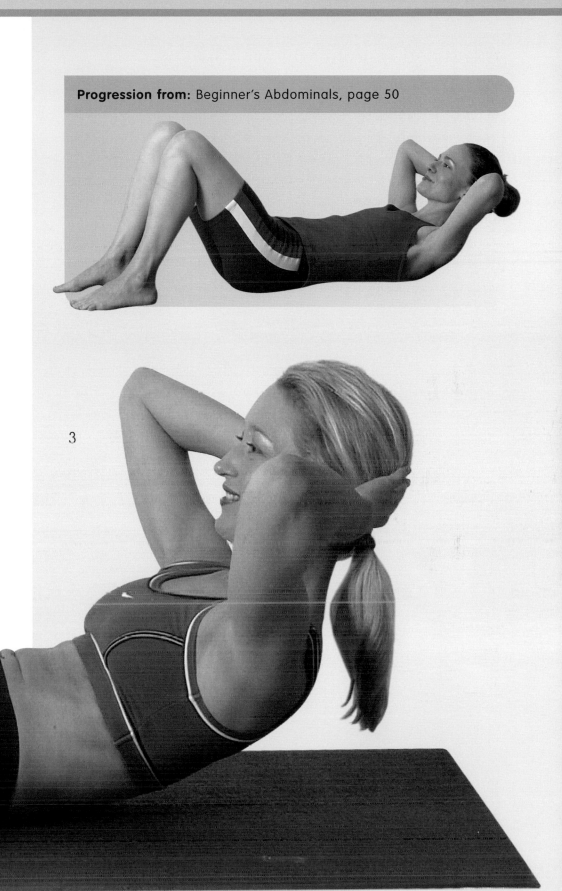

3

Advanced Abdominals with Twist

The Advanced Abdominals with Twist isolates the various muscles of the abdominals. The rectus abdominals support the spine, while the obliques flex, rotate and side-bend the torso. Perform the exercise slowly and concentrate on lengthening the abdominals down. If the stomach pops out you are coming up too high!

1 Lie on your back with your knees bent and your feet hip-width apart. Lace the fingers behind your head and slightly lift your elbows off the mat. Take a breath, inhaling.

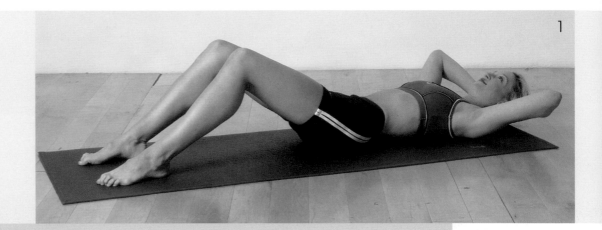

2 As you exhale, slowly pull the navel into the spine as you curl the upper torso forwards. Stay exactly where you are in space and take a breath, inhaling.

3 Exhale, leave the hips square and twist your upper torso towards the left. Try to keep both shoulder blades off the mat.

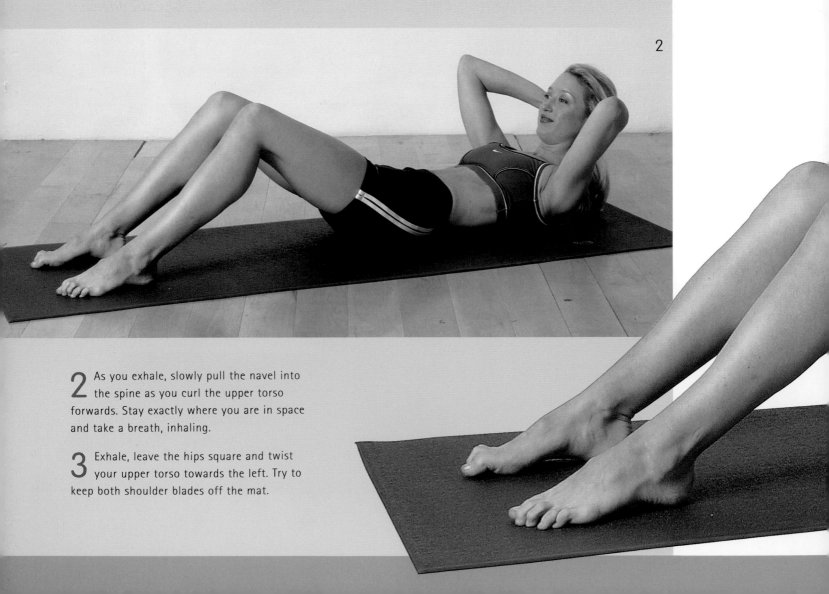

4 Inhale and relax the upper torso back on the mat.

5 Repeat immediately on the other side.

6 Repeat the whole exercise five times.

Key Points:

- Relax your neck, rest your head back in the hands and let your arms lift your head up.

- Try not to rest on your shoulders.

- Think of lifting both shoulder blades off the floor as you curl forwards.

- Keep the feet and knees hip-width apart.

- Pull the shoulder blades down the back.

- Keep the navel pulling into your spine and breathe through the sides and back of the ribs.

- Do not tuck the pelvis as you curl forwards.

Progression from: Obliques, page 52

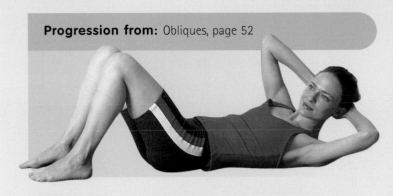

Challenge:

Criss Cross, page 164

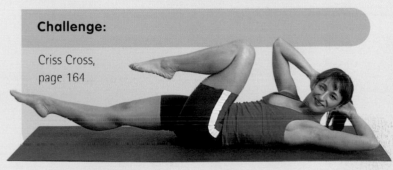

3

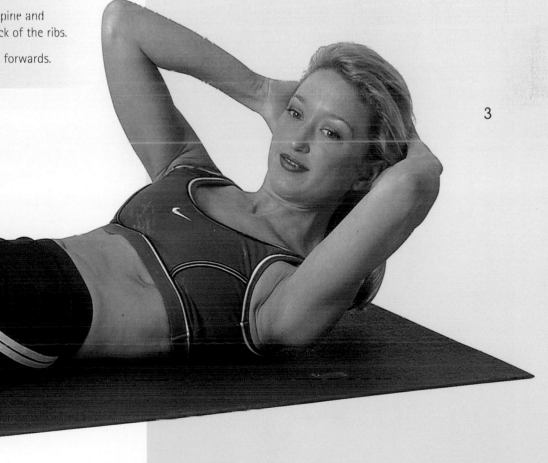

Leg Lifts

The Leg Lifts are designed to strengthen the muscles on the front of the thigh and their attachments, the quadriceps and hip flexors.

1 Sit on the floor with your back flat against a wall and your legs out straight. Relax your arms down by your sides and breathe naturally for the whole of the exercise.

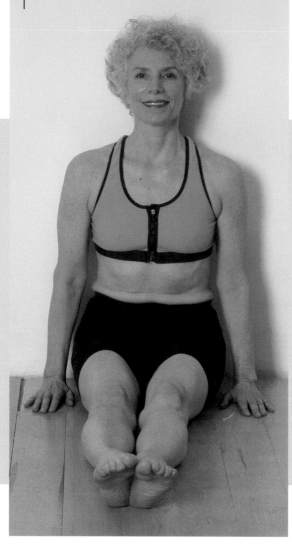

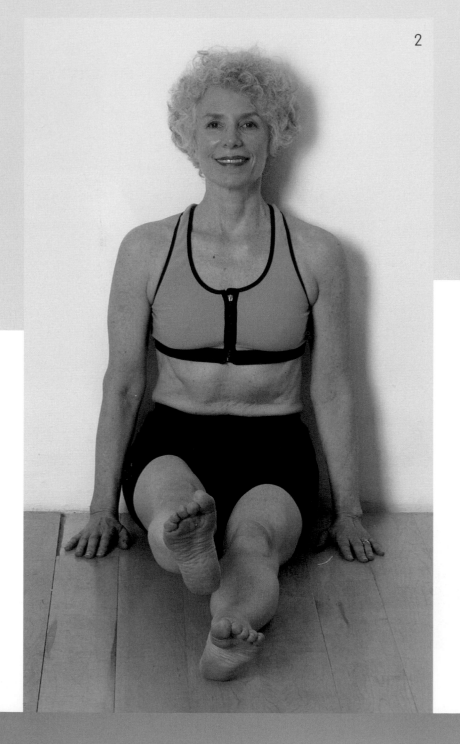

2 Lift your right leg 5cm/2in. off the floor. Hold for a slow count of five.

3 Keeping the right leg in the air, move the leg to the right without changing your hips. Hold for another slow count of five.

4 Still keeping the leg 5cm/2in off the ground, move the leg back in front of you for the last slow count of five.

5 Relax and repeat immediately on the other side.

6 Repeat each leg three times.

3

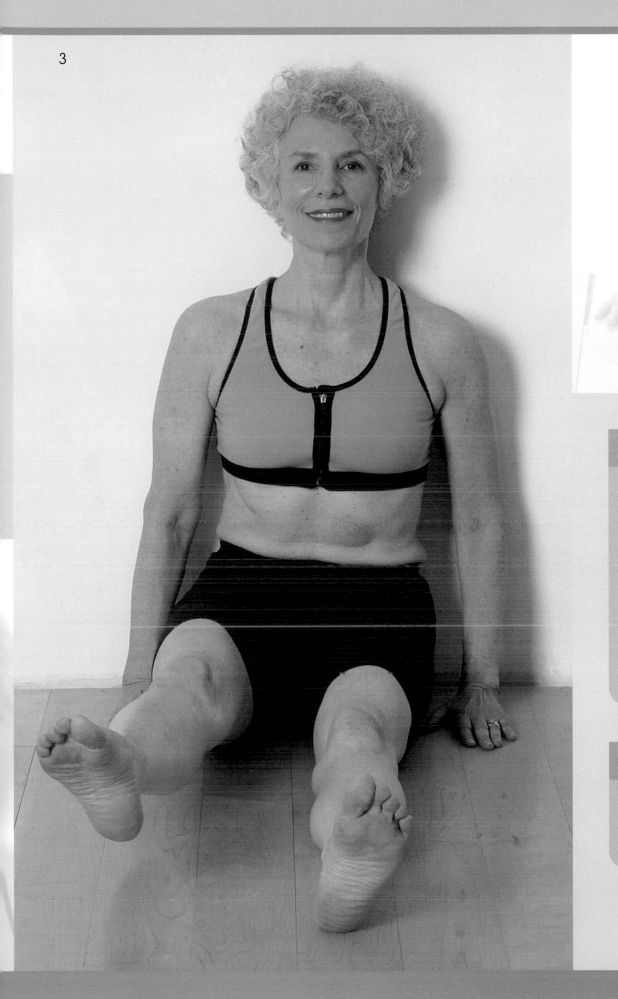

Key Points:

- Make sure the shoulders do not rise up.

- Keep the hips square throughout the exercise.

- Keep the navel pulling into the spine and breathe through the sides and back of the ribs.

- Keep the knee and foot facing the ceiling.

Modification:

If this feels too difficult, move the pelvis slightly away from the wall.

Frog

Frog brings all of the isolations of the previous section together. This exercise is for co-ordination of movement. Concentrate on performing all of the various aspects of the exercise together in one fluid motion.

1 Lie on your back with your knees into your chest and your feet together. Your knees should be shoulder-width apart so that the knees and ankles form a V. Take a breath, inhaling.

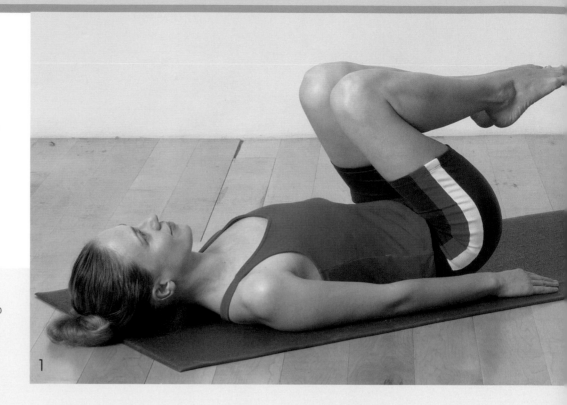

2 Lace your fingers behind your head and lift your elbows slightly off the mat. Take a breath, inhaling

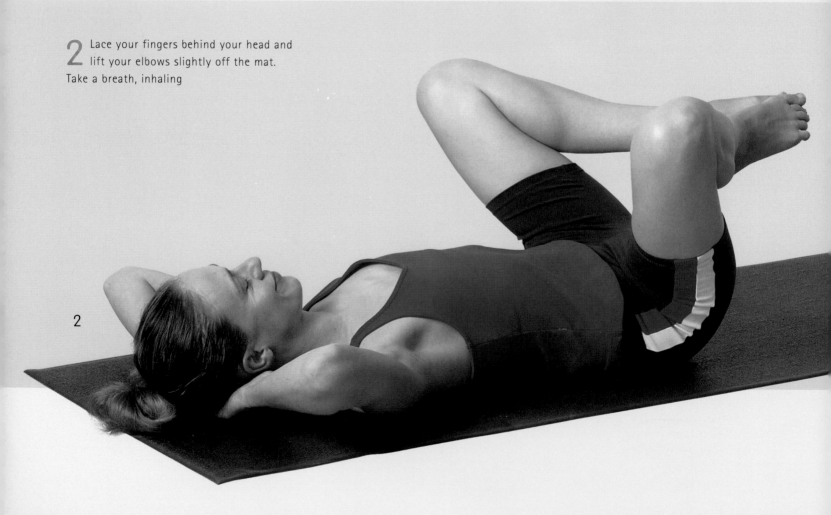

3 As you exhale, pull the navel into the spine and lift your head while extending the legs at a 45 degree angle.

4 Inhale to relax back to the starting position.

5 Repeat five times.

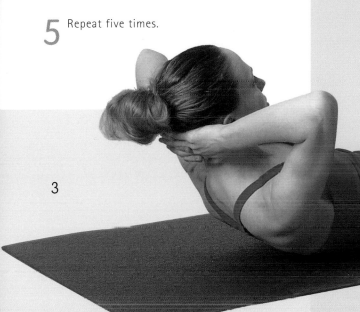

3

Key Points:

- Make sure your back does not arch.

- Keep the shoulder blades pulling down the back and your neck long.

- Relax your head back in your hands and lift the head with your arms.

- Squeeze the buttocks and inner thighs to support the lower back.

- Extend through your toes.

- Keep the navel pulling into your spine and breathe through the sides and back of your ribs.

Progression from:

Teaser with Feet on Chair, page 69.

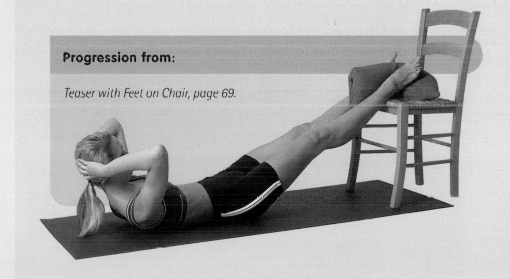

*This is an **adaptation**
*of an **original** PILATES
*exercise**

Elementary Hundred

The Elementary Hundred gets the blood pumping, increasing circulation and stamina.

1 Lie on your back with your knees bent all the way into the chest and your arms resting by your sides. Lift your feet up to the ceiling so that your hips and knees make a right angle. Squeeze your buttocks and inner thighs while lengthening out through your toes. Your back should be glued into the mat. Pull your shoulder blades down your back as you round forwards from the top of your head. Lift your head off the floor, place your chin into your chest and look at your navel. Lift your arms up so that they are parallel to the ground and straight.

2 Working from the abdominals, pump the arms vigorously up and down 8cm/3in. without letting them touch the mat.

3 Inhale for five pumps through the nose, and exhale through the mouth for five pumps.

4 Repeat ten times.

1

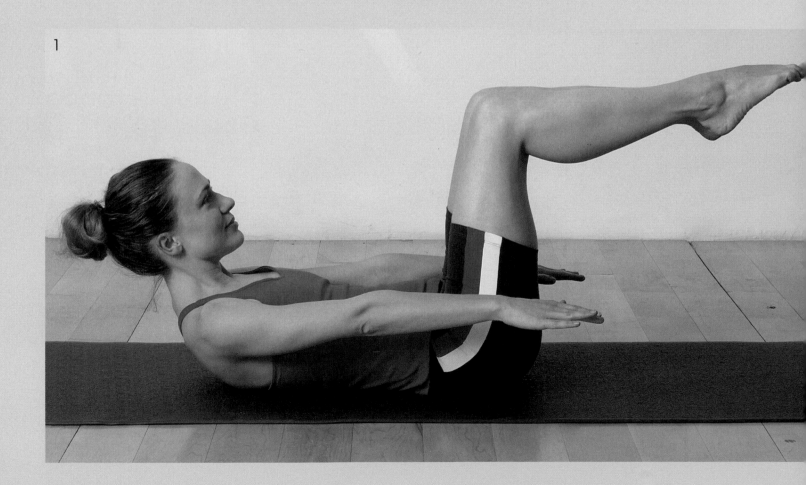

2

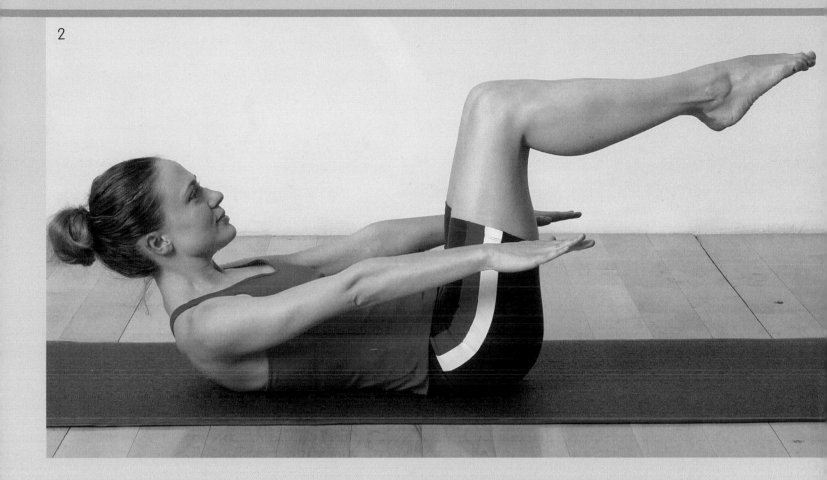

Key Points:

- Keep the shoulder blades pulling down the back.

- Keep the navel pulling into your spine and breathe through the sides and back of your ribs.

- Reach the fingertips long.

- Squeeze the buttocks and inner thighs to support the lower back.

- Extend through the toes.

*This is an **adaptation** of an **original** PILATES exercise*

Modification:

If you are feeling tension in the neck, relax the head for a few breaths and then pick the head back up to the original position.

Challenge: See the Hundred on page 144.

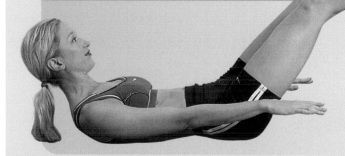

Basic Roll-up

This Basic Roll-up strengthens the abdominals while stretching the lower back and hamstrings.

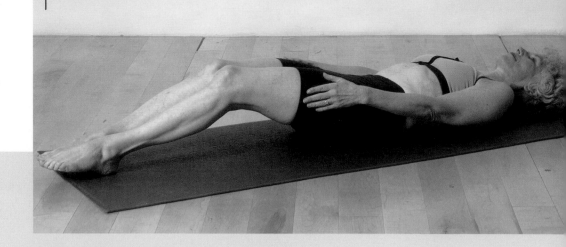

1 Lie on your back with your hands touching your thighs, knees slightly bent and glued together.

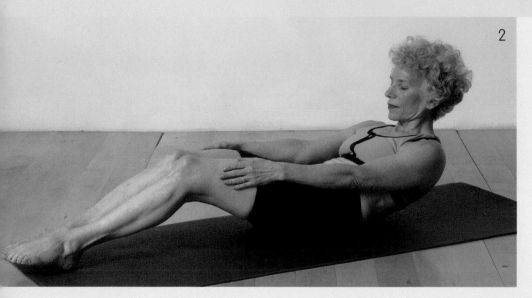

2 As you inhale, bring your chin into your chest and use your abdominals to curl each vertebra off the mat sequentially. If you are finding this difficult, hold on to your legs and bend your elbows out to the sides to help you roll up.

3 As you curl up to a sitting position, exhale and extend your legs and hold on to your ankles. Pull your head towards your knees, while keeping your shoulders down. This will stretch out the lower back and hamstrings.

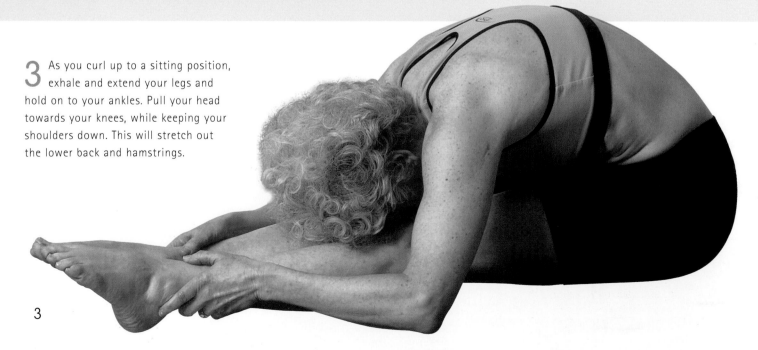

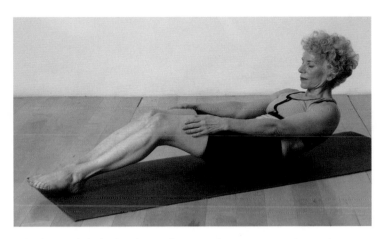

4 As you inhale, bend your knees and squeeze your buttocks as you round backwards, vertebra by vertebra.

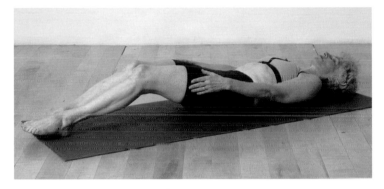

5 Exhale to relax.

6 Repeat five times.

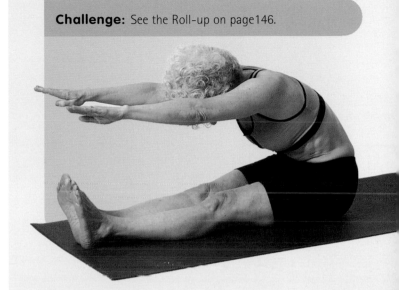

Challenge: See the Roll-up on page146.

*This is an **adaptation** *of an* **original** PILATES *exercise*

Key Points:

- Make sure your back is rounding and not arching.

- Keep the shoulder blades pulling down the back.

- Squeeze the inner thighs and buttocks as you roll up and down to support the lower back.

- Keep the navel pulling into your spine and breathe through the sides and back of your ribs.

Hamstring Stretch

The Hamstring Stretch lengthens the back of the leg while maintaining form and alignment.

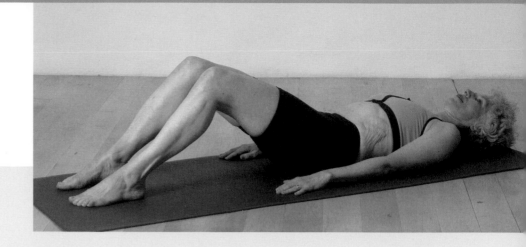

1 Lie on your back with your knees bent and your feet hip-width apart

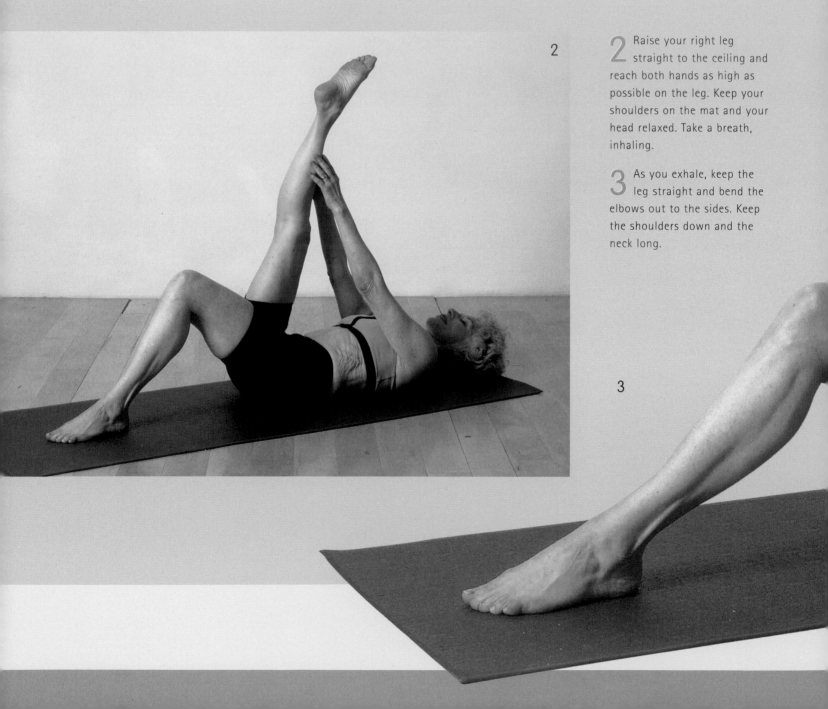

2

2 Raise your right leg straight to the ceiling and reach both hands as high as possible on the leg. Keep your shoulders on the mat and your head relaxed. Take a breath, inhaling.

3 As you exhale, keep the leg straight and bend the elbows out to the sides. Keep the shoulders down and the neck long.

3

Key Points:

- Extend through your toes to the ceiling.

- Keep your shoulder blades pulling down your back.

- Press your elbows to the sides so that you feel your biceps working.

- Do not let your pelvis come off the mat.

4 Inhale and relax the elbows.

5 Repeat three times.

6 Repeat on the other side.

Progression from:

Hamstring Stretch Sitting, page 46

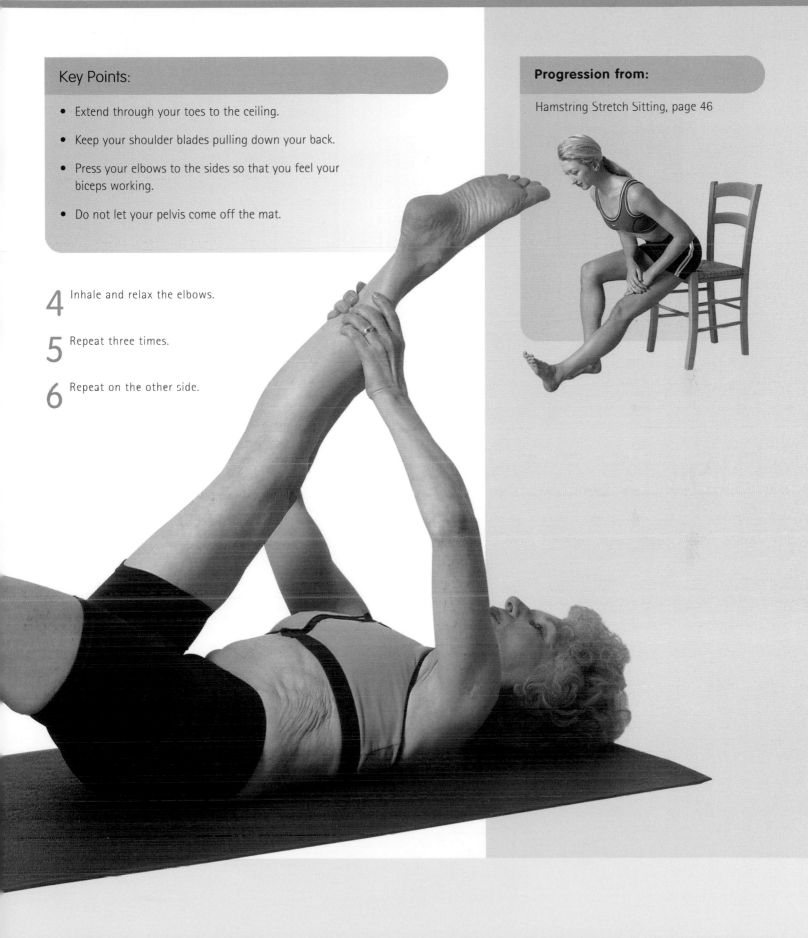

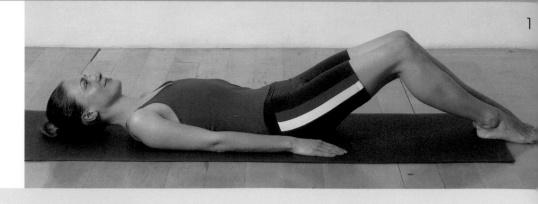

Basic Leg Circles

This exercise works on stretching the legs and increasing hip mobility while initiating the movement with the abdominals.

1 Lie down on the mat with your knees slightly bent and your feet hip-width apart. Relax your arms down by your sides.

2 Bend the left leg slightly and extend it towards the ceiling. Focus on moving the leg with the breath.

3 As you inhale, cross the left leg over the midline of the body, initiating a circle.

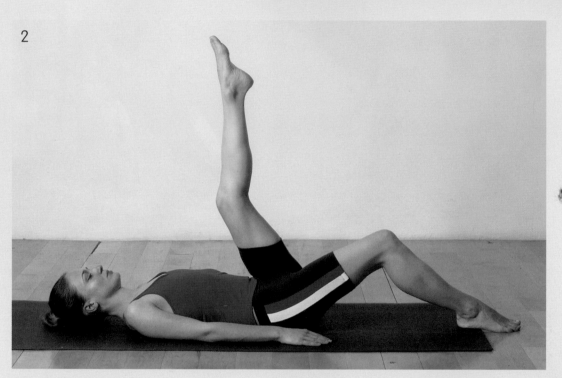

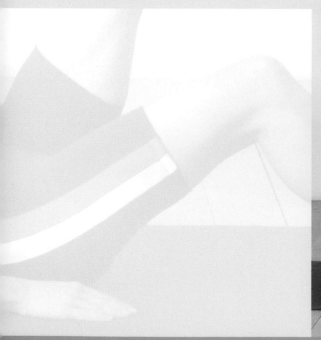

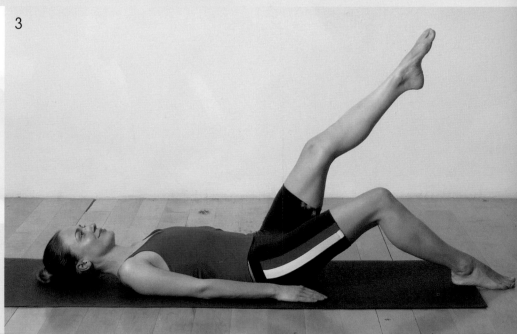

4 As you exhale, complete the second half of the circle and pull your navel down into your spine. You want to be thinking of touching your nose with your foot.

5 Repeat five times in this direction, and then reverse directions.

4

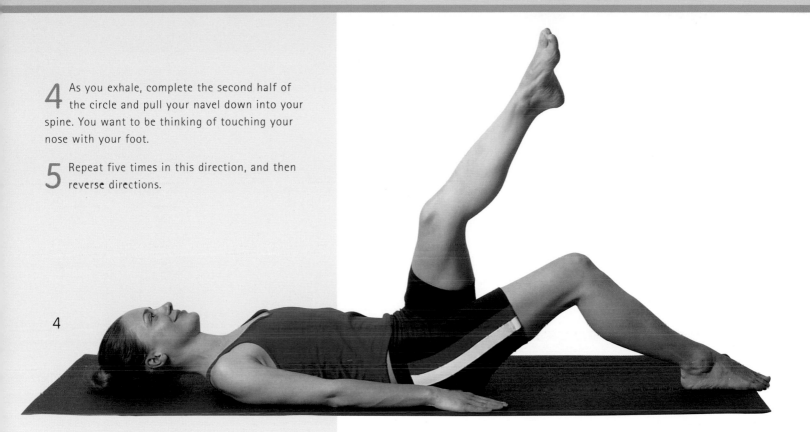

Key Points:

- Make sure the hips stay square the whole time.

- Pull your shoulder blades down your back.

- Press your hands into the floor to help stabilize.

- Accent is on the upswing towards your nose.

- Keep the navel pulling into your spine and breathe through the sides and back of your ribs.

*This is an **adaptation** *of an* **original** PILATES *exercise**

Progression from:

Abdominal Isolation, page 59

Challenge:

Leg Circles, page 151

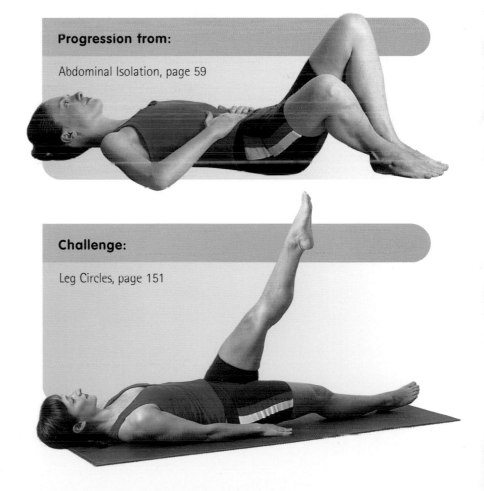

Rolling Like a Ball Open

This exercise focuses on balance, co-ordination, strengthening your powerhouse and mobilizing your back.

1 Sit up with the soles of the feet together and the knees bent out to the sides, shoulder-width apart. Hold on to the undersides of your knees and lift your feet off the floor. Round your back and drop your chin into your chest. You should be balancing on your pelvis.

2 As you inhale, pull the navel into your spine and round your tailbone underneath you. Roll backwards on to your shoulders and let your pelvis float into the air.

3 Exhale and roll back up to a sitting position without letting your feet touch the ground.

4 Repeat four to eight times.

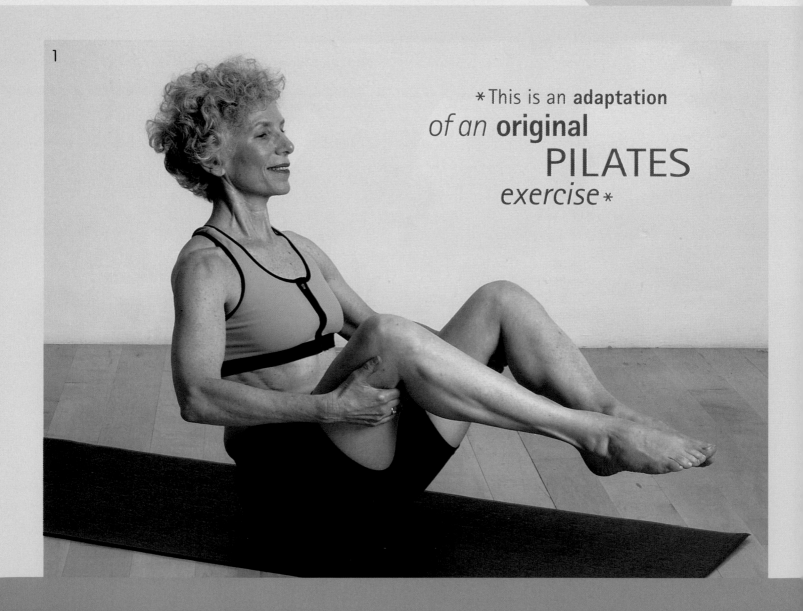

1

*This is an **adaptation** of an **original** PILATES exercise*

2

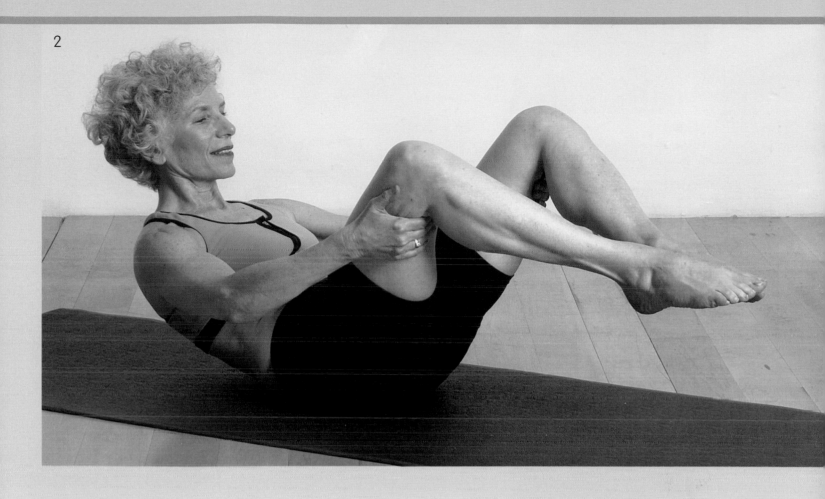

Key Points:

- Only roll back to the shoulder blades.
- Keep the navel pulling into your spine and breathe through the sides and back of your ribs.
- Keep the shoulder blades down and the elbows out to the sides.
- Do not use momentum and try not to use your legs or hip flexors.

Challenge:

See Rolling Like a Ball on page154.

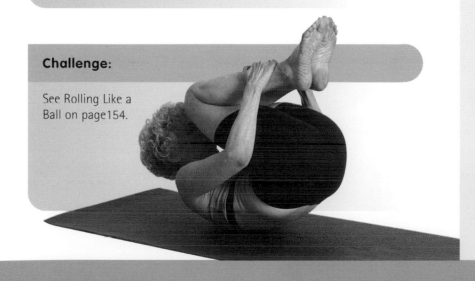

Progression from:

Pelvic Curl , page 48

Cat, page 56

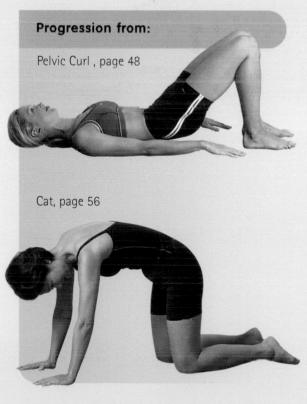

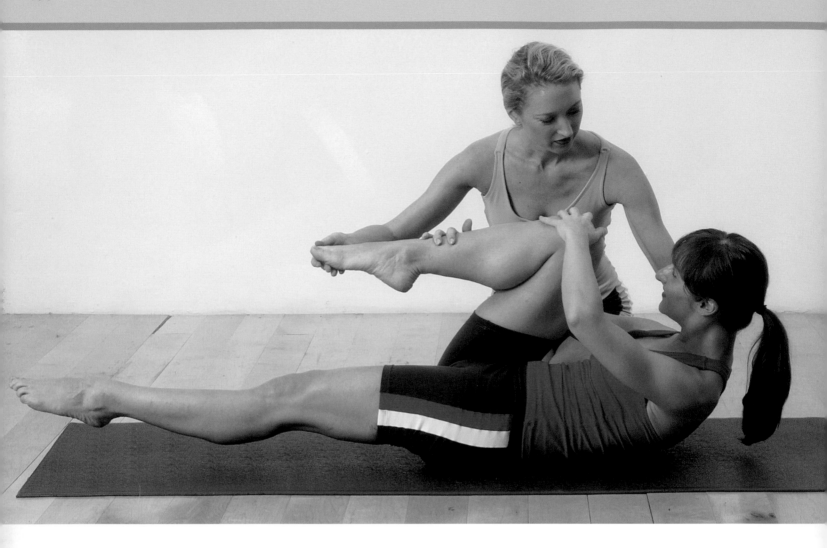

Elementary Single Leg Stretch

The Elementary Single Leg Stretch is a precursor to the Single Leg Stretch (page 156) shown here. It is important to perform this exercise slowly, focusing on co-ordinating all the various aspects of the movements.

1 Hold on with both hands to the underside of your right thigh, and lift your head and shoulders off the mat. Lift your left leg off the ground and squeeze your buttocks as you reach the toes out long. Take a breath, inhaling.

2 As you exhale, pull the navel further down into the mat and pull your elbows out to the sides. Make sure the shoulder blades are down on the back.

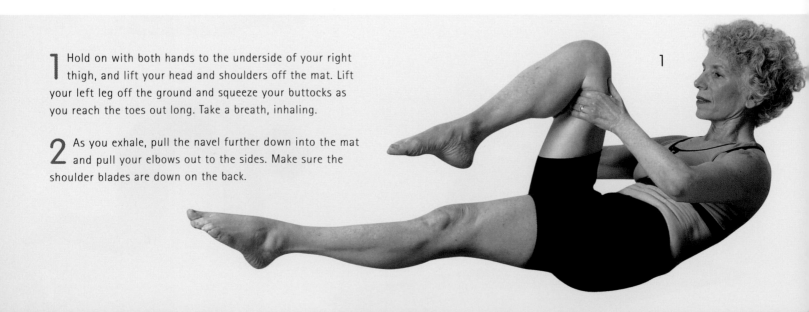

3 Keeping your upper torso where it is, inhale and change your legs.

4 Exhale and pull the abdominals further down as you hold on to the left leg.

5 Repeat each leg five times.

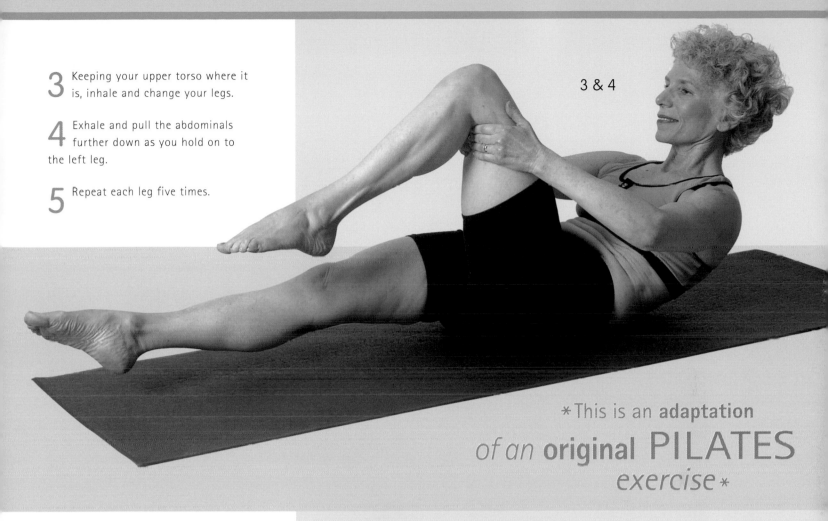

3 & 4

*This is an **adaptation**
of an **original** PILATES
exercise *

Key Points:

- Keep the neck relaxed and the abdominals engaged.

- Keep the navel pulling into your spine and breathe through the sides and back of your ribs.

- Keep the shoulder blades pulling down the back.

- Squeeze the buttocks and lengthen through your toes.

- Press your elbows out to the side walls.

Challenge:

Single Leg Stretch, page 156

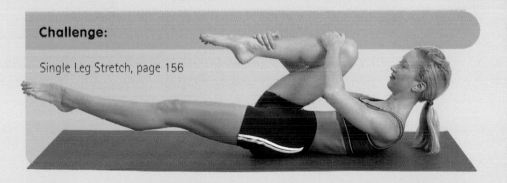

Progression from:

Abdominals with Arm Extension , page 60

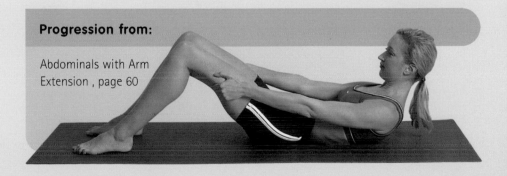

Single Straight Leg Stretch

The Single Straight Leg Stretch focuses on strengthening the abdominals and stretching the hamstrings.

1 Lie on your back with your legs extended straight towards the ceiling.

2 Grasp your left leg with both hands as high up towards the ankle as you can comfortably hold. Extend the right leg so that it is hovering 5cm/2in. off the floor. Raise your chin to your chest and drop your shoulders down your back. Pull the straight right leg towards your head and pulse twice.

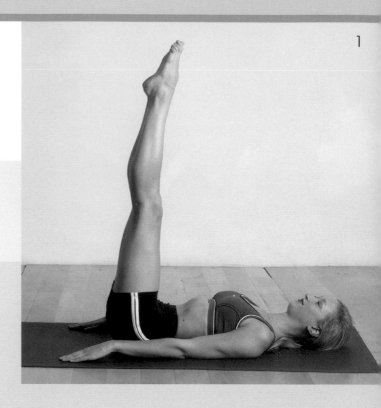

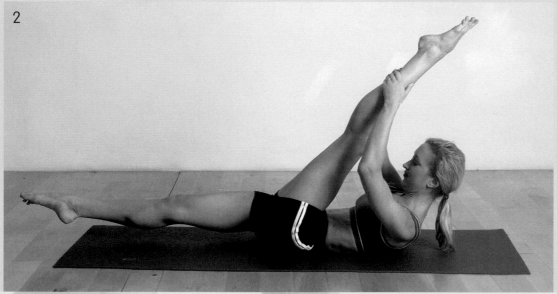

3 Switch the legs, keeping them straight, and pulse twice with the right.

4 Inhale for one set, and exhale for another.

5 Counting your right and left leg as one, repeat five to ten times.

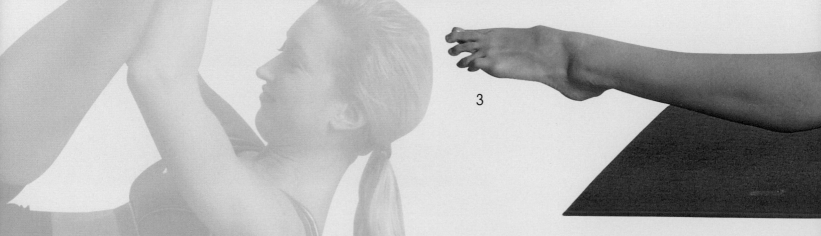

Key Points:

- Keep the shoulder blades pulling down the back.

- Keep the neck long.

- Pull your elbows out to the side walls.

- Keep the navel pulling into your spine and breathe through the sides and back of your ribs.

- Keep the legs straight and reach out with your toes.

Modification:

If the neck gets tired, place the head down and keep going.

*This is an
original
PILATES
exercise*

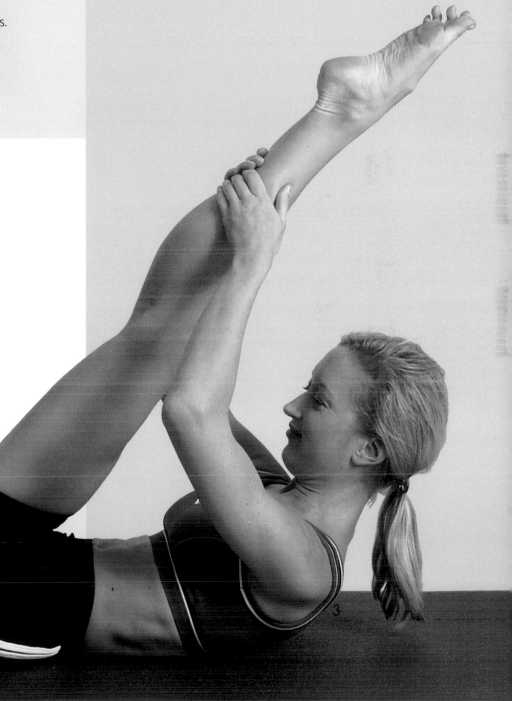

Double Bent Leg Stretch

The Double Bent Leg Stretch is a precursor to the Double Straight Leg Stretch found in the next section. This exercise strengthens your abdominals while continuing to isolate the legs moving from the powerhouse.

1 Lie down with your hands under the lower part of your pelvis, palms facing downwards. This cradles the lower back into the floor. Bend your knees into your chest and slightly extend the legs towards the ceiling. Keep your head relaxed down at all times.

1

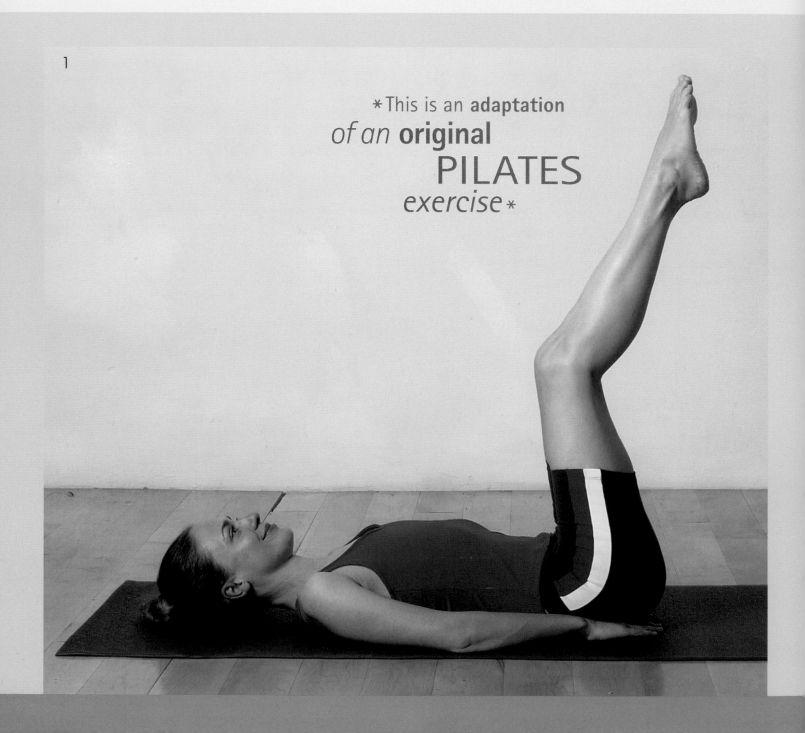

*This is an **adaptation** *of an* **original** PILATES *exercise*∗

2

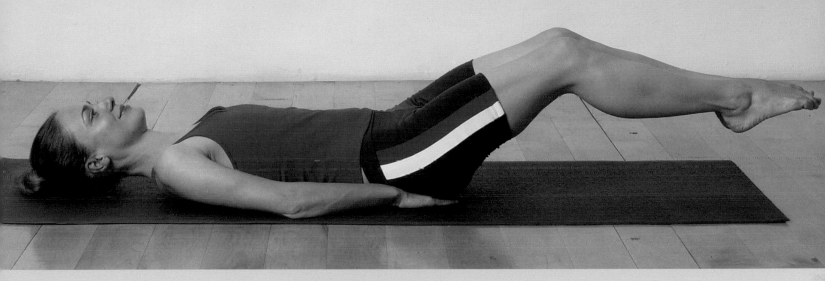

2 As you inhale, lower the toes down towards the mat without changing your spine.

3 As you exhale, pull the navel into the mat and lift the legs back to their starting position

4 Repeat ten times.

Key Points:

- Make sure the back stays flat the whole time.
- Keep your shoulder blades pulling down your back.
- Keep the navel pulling into your spine and breathe through the sides and back of your ribs.
- Squeeze your inner thighs and buttocks to support your lower spine.

Challenge: Double Straight Leg Stretch, page 162

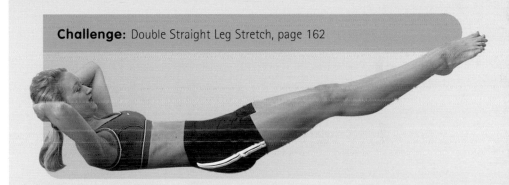

Progression from:

Single Leg Lifts, page 62

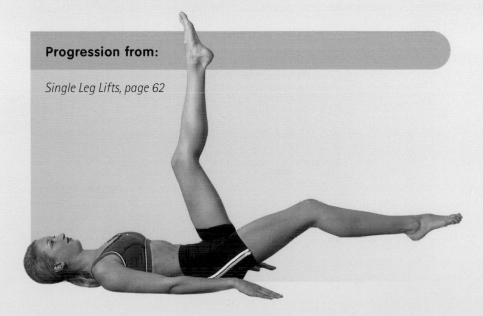

Criss Cross

The Criss Cross focuses on co-ordination and abdominal strength, especially the obliques. Think of moving fluidly from your powerhouse.

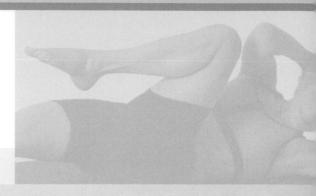

1

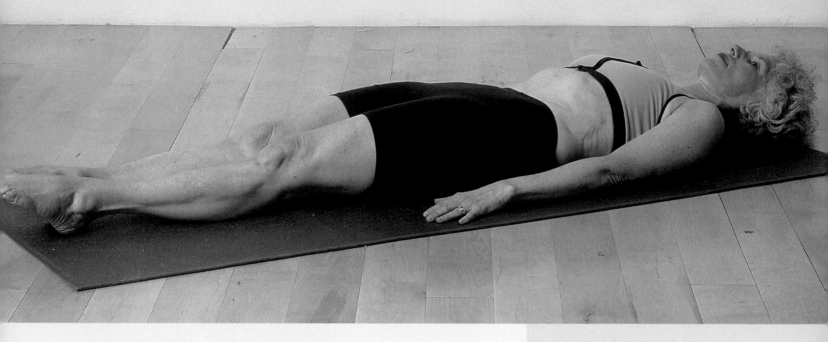

1 Lie on your back with your legs extended along the mat and your arms down by your side.

2 Bend your left knee into your chest and lift your left leg to a 45-degree angle off the ground. Lace the fingers behind your head.As you inhale, twist towards the left so that the right elbow is touching the left knee. Look over your left shoulder. Hold for three counts.

3 As you exhale, twist to the other side, bringing your right knee into the chest and extending the left leg out long. Look over your right shoulder.

2

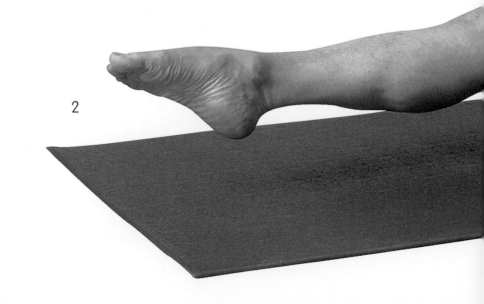

Key Points:

- Make sure the legs do not go out to the sides but stay directly in line with your hips.

- Keep the navel pulling into your spine and breathe through the sides and back of your ribs.

- Keep your shoulder blades down and twist from the waistline.

- Look behind you on the twist, keeping the shoulders open.

- Do not twist in the hips. Keep them glued to the floor.

4 Inhale as you hold for another three counts.

5 Repeat for five times each side.

Progression from:

Obliques, page 52.

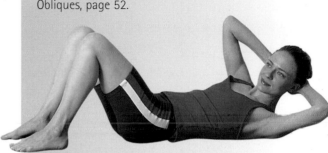

*This is an
original PILATES
exercise *

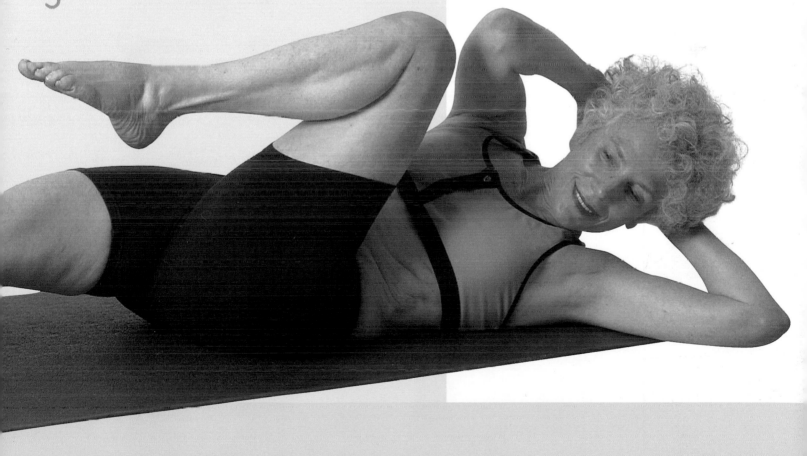

Spine Stretch Forward

The Spine Stretch Forward is great for posture and breathing. It also strengthens the abdominals while stretching the middle and lower back.

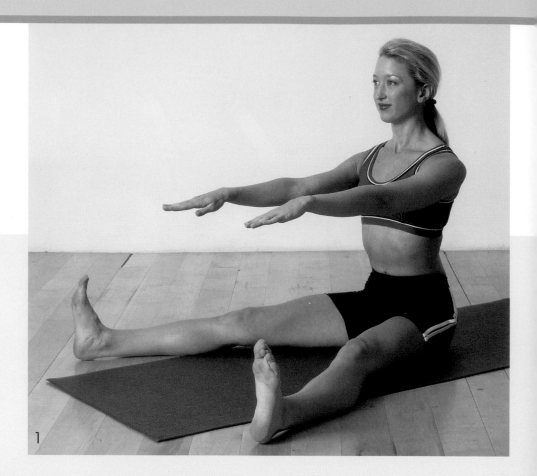

1 Sit up on the mat with your legs out straight just a little more than shoulder-width apart, and your arms extended out in front of you parallel to the ground. Take a breath, inhaling.

2 As you exhale, pull your shoulder blades down and round forwards, starting from the top of your head and keeping your arms straight out in front of you.

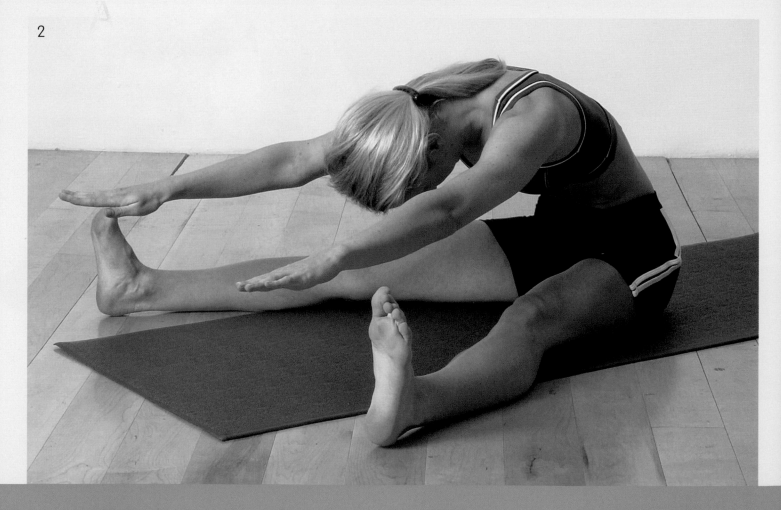

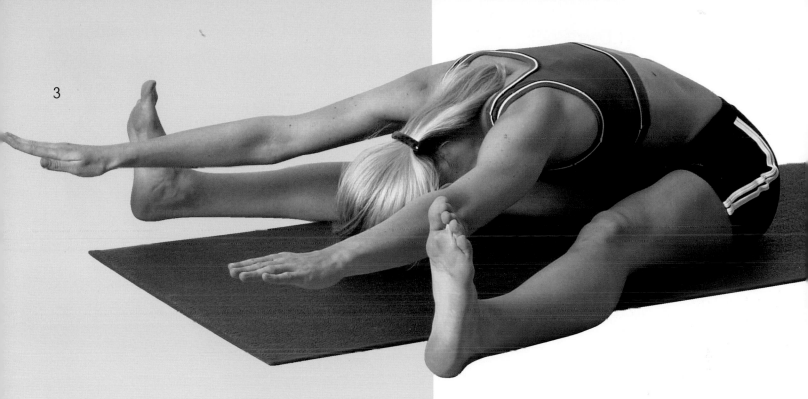

3

3 Think of rounding over a big ball in front of you. You want to keep the stomach engaged and the tailbone down on the mat.

4 Inhale to roll back up to a sitting position.

5 Repeat five times.

*This is an
original PILATES
*exercise**

Key Points:

- Make sure the back is long and tall in the starting position. You might need to sit up on a firm pillow or bend your knees slightly.

- Keep the pelvis anchored into the floor.

- Keep your shoulder blades pulling down your back.

- Keep the navel pulling into your spine and breathe through the sides and back of your ribs.

- Think of rolling sequentially through your spine.

Progression from: The Cat, page 57.

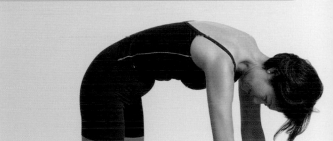

Prep for Open Leg Rocker

The main objective of this exercise is to find your balance and co-ordination in order to perform advanced exercises more precisely. Focus on finding your balance on your tailbone, while moving the limbs easily from the powerhouse.

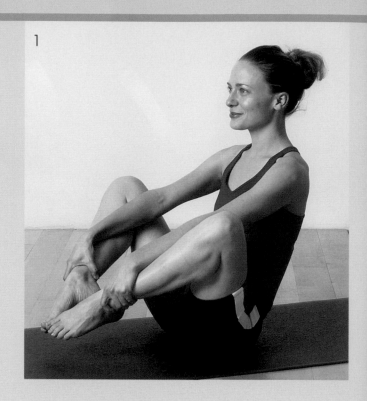

1 Sit up on the mat. Bend your knees and hold on to your ankles with your arms on the inside of your knees. Lift your feet and balance on your tailbone. Take a breath, inhaling.

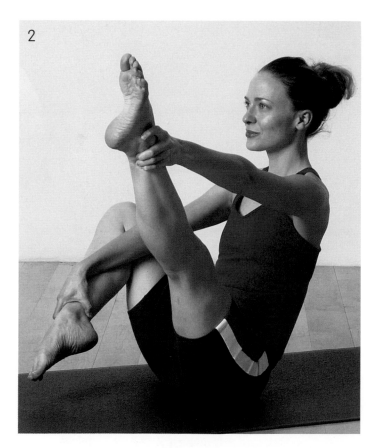

2 As you exhale, extend your left knee and arm towards your left shoulder. Make sure you do not raise the shoulder with the leg.

3 As you inhale, bend the leg back to the original position without letting the foot touch the ground.

4 As you exhale for the second time, extend the right leg towards the right shoulder.

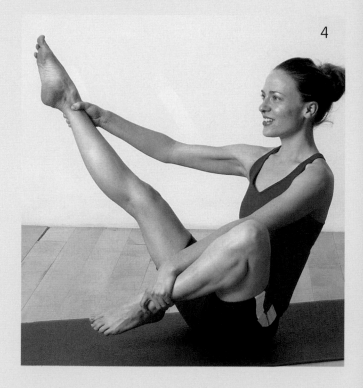

5 As you inhale, bend the leg back into the original position.

6 On the third exhale, try extending both legs at the same time without losing your balance.

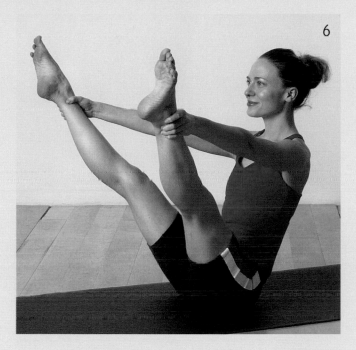

6

7 As you inhale, keep the legs straight and bring them together.

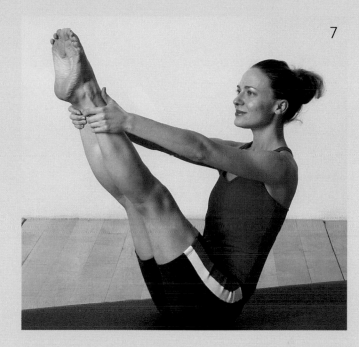

7

8 As you exhale, keep the legs straight and open them back out to shoulder-width.

9 Inhale to relax.

10 Repeat three times.

Key Points:

- Make sure you stay up on your tailbone so that you do not fall backwards.

- Keep the navel pulling into your spine and breathe through the sides and back of your ribs.

- Keep your shoulder blades pulling down your back.

- Extend through your toes.

Challenge:

Open Leg Rocker, page 168.

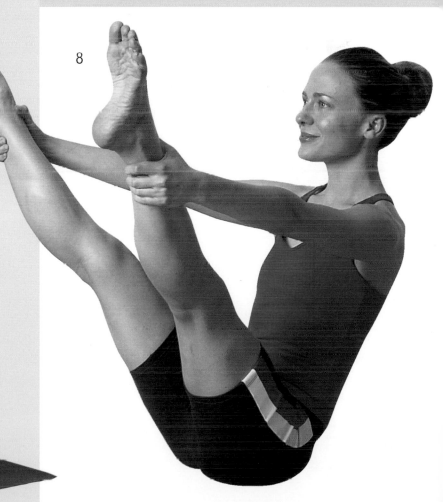

8

Tick Tock

The Tick Tock focuses on stretching and strengthening the torso, legs and hips.

1 Lie on your back with your arms extended straight out to the sides at shoulder level, palms facing upwards. Raise your legs to the ceiling, trying to keep them as straight as possible. Toes apart, heels together.

2 As you inhale, lower the legs towards your left side, keeping them at a right angle to your torso.

3 As you exhale, pull the navel down towards the spine and lift the legs back to the original position.

4 On your next inhale, lower the legs towards your right side, again keeping them at a right angle to your torso.

5 On your next exhale, pull the navel down towards the spine and lift the legs back to the original position.

6 Repeat four times to each side.

1

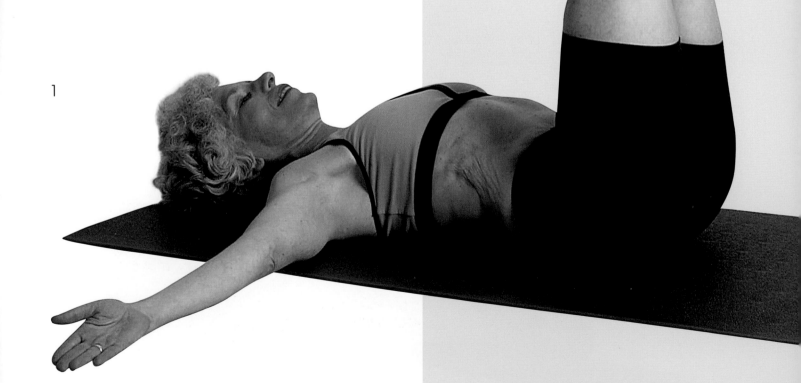

2

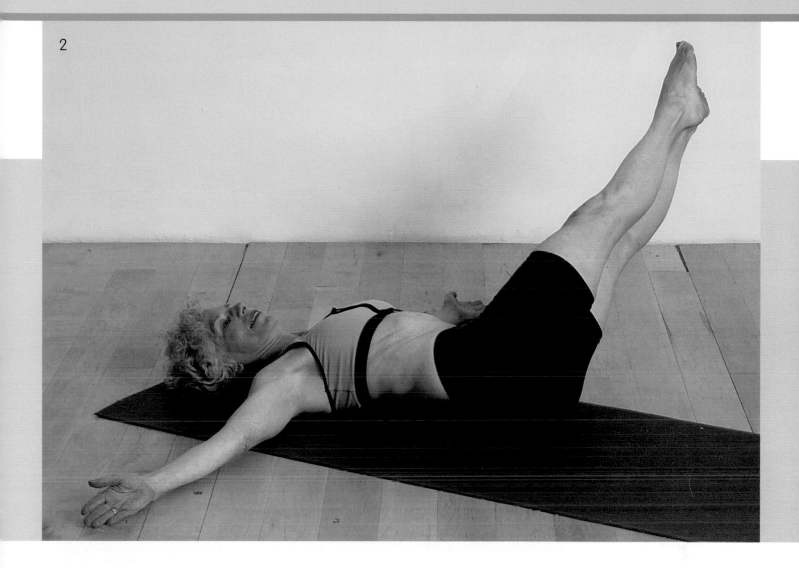

Key Points:

- Press your hands into the floor for stabilization.

- Twist from the waistline.

- Squeeze your inner thighs and buttocks together to help support the lower back.

- Keep the navel pulling into your spine and breathe through the sides and back of your ribs.

- Do not let the shoulders come off the floor.

*This is an
original
PILATES
*exercise**

Modification:

If this exercise feels difficult, bend the knees slightly, keeping feet parallel.

Pelvic Lifts
Ankles Crossed

The purpose of this exercise is to find the connection between the stomach and the buttocks. It works the backs of the arms as well.

1

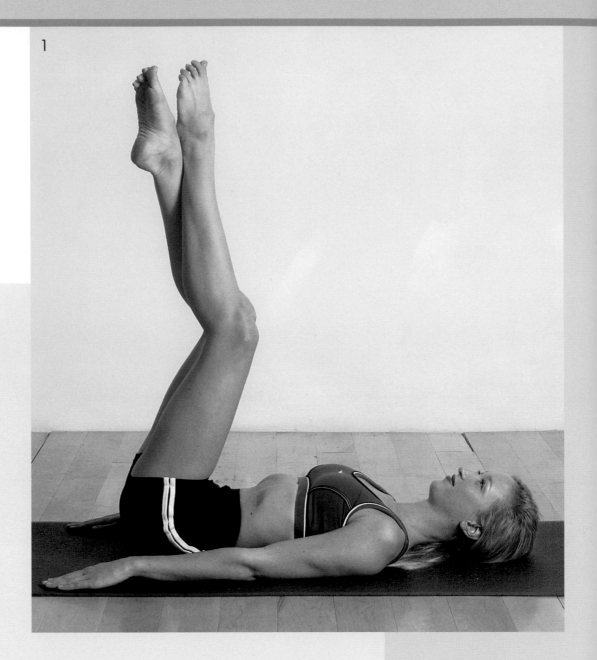

1 Lie on your back with your feet in the air and your ankles crossed. Lengthen your arms down by your sides. Take a breath, inhaling.

2 As you exhale, press the arms down into the mat. Move the knees slightly forwards and into the chest. As you do this, pinch your buttocks and lift the pelvis off the mat.

3 Inhale to relax.

4 Repeat three to five times.

Key Points:

- If you feel any tension in the lower back, please leave this exercise out.

- Keep the shoulder blades pulling down the back.

- Make sure you relax the head and neck.

- Press the hands into the floor to help the buttocks lift off the mat.

- Keep the navel pulling into your spine and breathe through the sides and back of your ribs.

- Only roll on to your shoulders, not the neck.

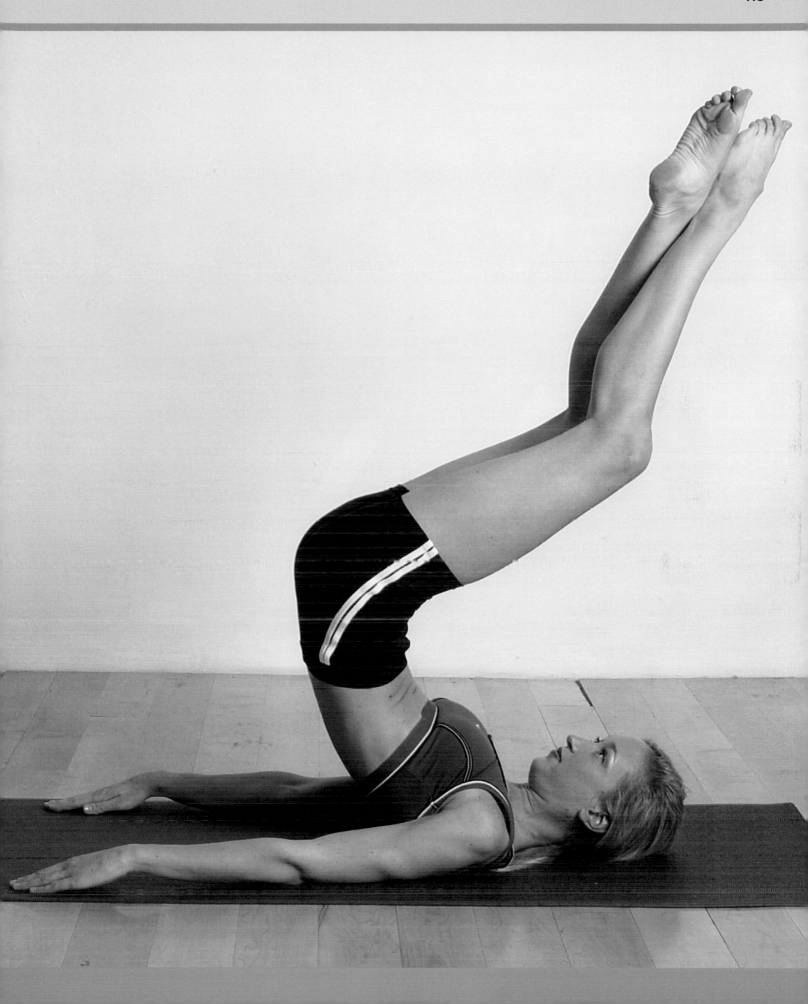

Small Corkscrew

The Small Corkscrew works on strengthening the abdominals, thigh muscles and hip flexors.

1 Lie on your back with your arms resting down by the sides of your body. Raise your legs straight up to the ceiling, toes apart and heels together.

2 Keeping the pelvis flat, imagine you are drawing circles on the ceiling with your toes. Inhale as your legs go towards the right and extend away from the body. Exhale as they circle to the left and back up to the original starting position.

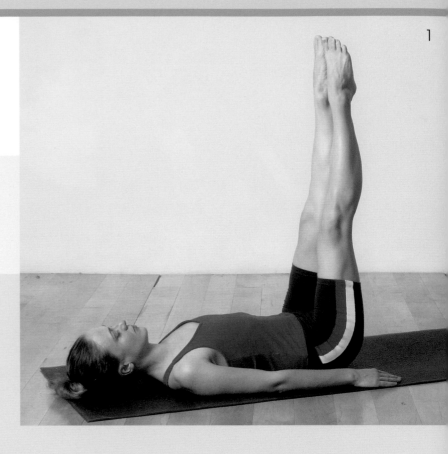

2

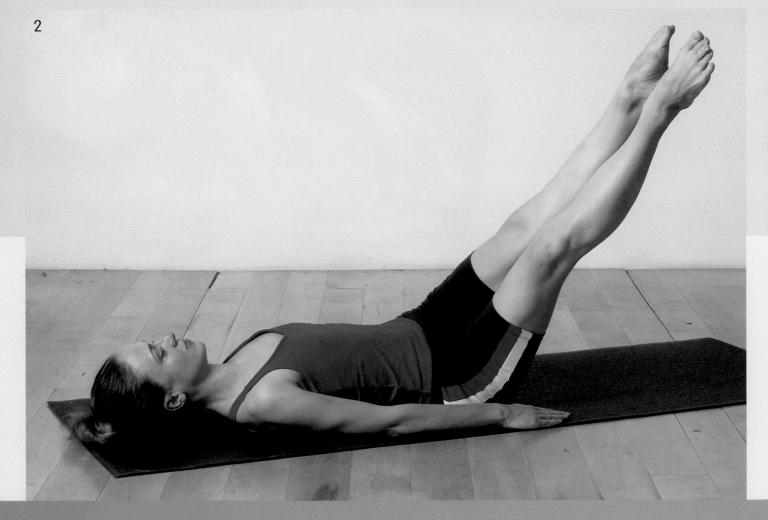

3 Immediately switch directions. Inhale as your legs lower to the left and away from the body, exhale as they circle to the right and back to the original starting position.

4 Keep the circles small.

5 Repeat four times on each side.

*This is an **adaptation** of an **original** PILATES exercise*

Key Points:

- Make sure the back does not arch on this exercise. Keep the circles as small as you need to and initiate the control of movement from the stomach.

- Keep the navel pulling into your spine and breathe through the sides and back of your ribs.

- Keep the shoulder blades pulling down your back.

- Press your hands into the floor for stabilization.

3

Modification:

Place the hands under the hips with the palms facing down. Bring the legs into parallel and bend the knees slightly. Keep the pelvis on the mat and make small circles.

Challenge:

Corkscrew, page 171

Saw

The Saw is a great exercise for stretching the inner thighs and hamstrings, strengthening the abdominals and articulating the back.

1 Sit up on your tailbone so that your back is flat and tall, legs straight out in front of you, just outside shoulder-width apart, and extend your arms out to the sides.

2 Inhale as you twist towards the left, pointing your right hand towards the left foot.

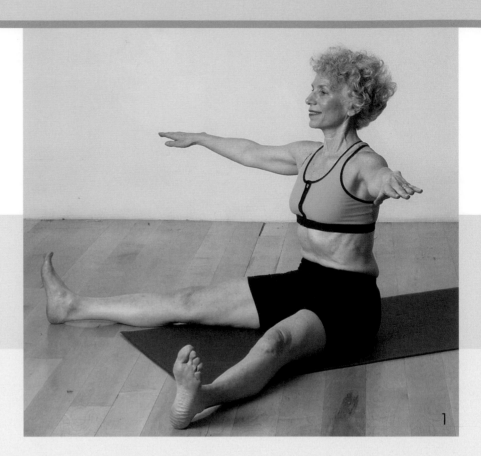

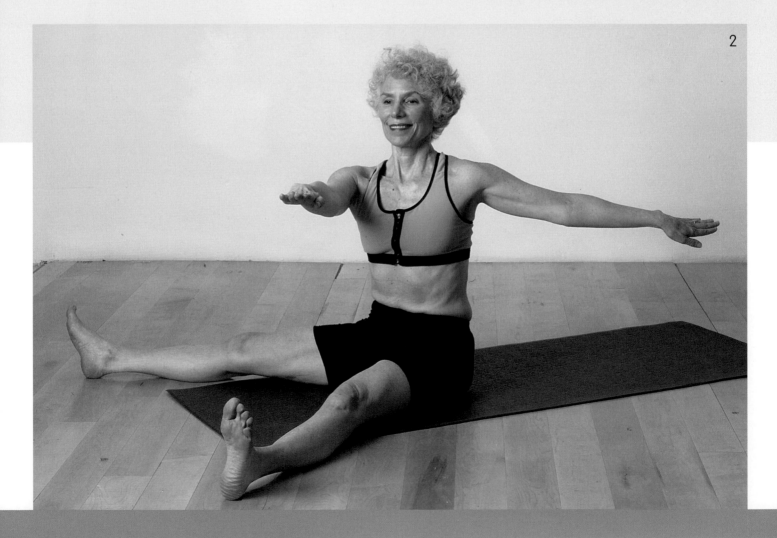

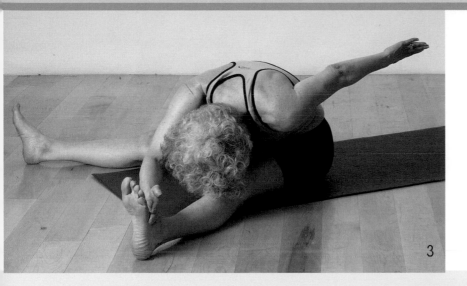

3

3 As you exhale, roll the top of your head towards your left knee and slide your right little finger to the outside of your left toes.

4 Inhale and roll back to the original position and start twisting to the right side. Exhale rolling down to the right knee with your left hand sawing past the right toes.

5 Repeat four times on each side.

4

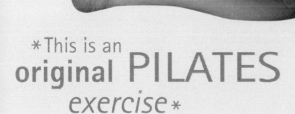

*This is an
original PILATES
exercise *

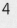

Key Points:

- Make sure the hips stay anchored into the ground.

- Keep the navel pulling into your spine and breathe through the sides and back of your ribs.

- Lengthen your head away from your tailbone.

- Extend through the arms and lengthen your fingertips.

Modification:

If you are finding this exercise difficult, you can bend your knees or sit on a firm cushion.

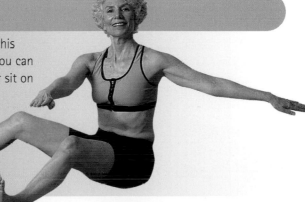

Spine Twist Knees Bent

The Spine Twist is the next progression of the Beginner's Twist on page44. It focuses on lengthening and stretching the spine while wringing out the lungs. Think of lifting the ribcage away from the hips while keeping the back long and pulling the shoulder blades down.

1 Sit up tall and slightly bend the knees, squeezing them tight together in front of you. Flex the feet. Reach your arms directly out to the sides. Think of lifting your chest and pulling your shoulders down, while keeping the ribcage in. Inhale to prepare.

2 As you exhale, twist to the left and pulse twice with your torso. Your hips should stay completely still. You want to think of pulling your shoulder blades down and opening your chest.

3 Face the front and inhale, while lengthening the head towards the ceiling.

4 On your next exhale, twist to the right and pulse twice.

5 Repeat four times on each side.

*This is an
original
PILATES
exercise*

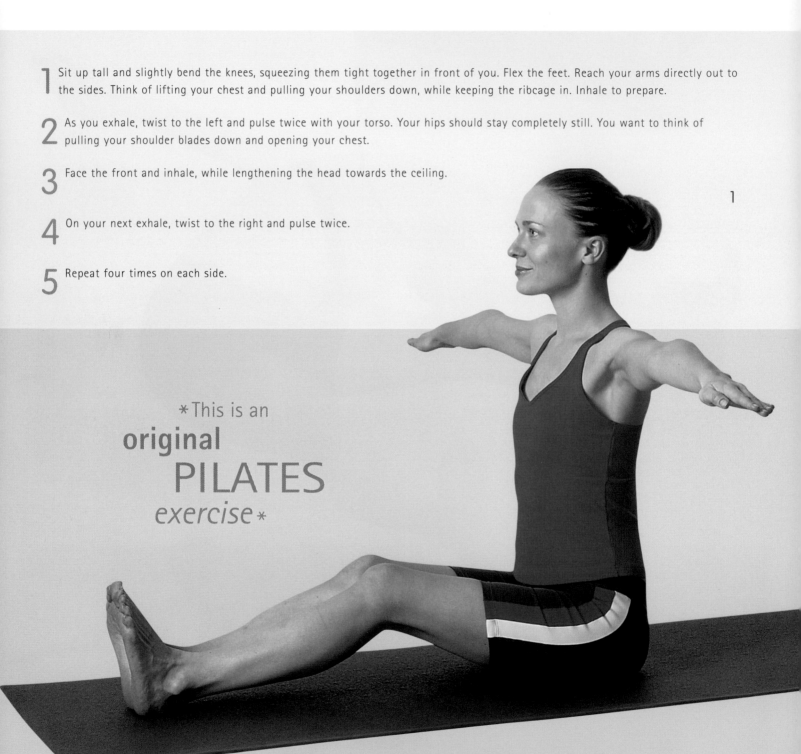

1

2

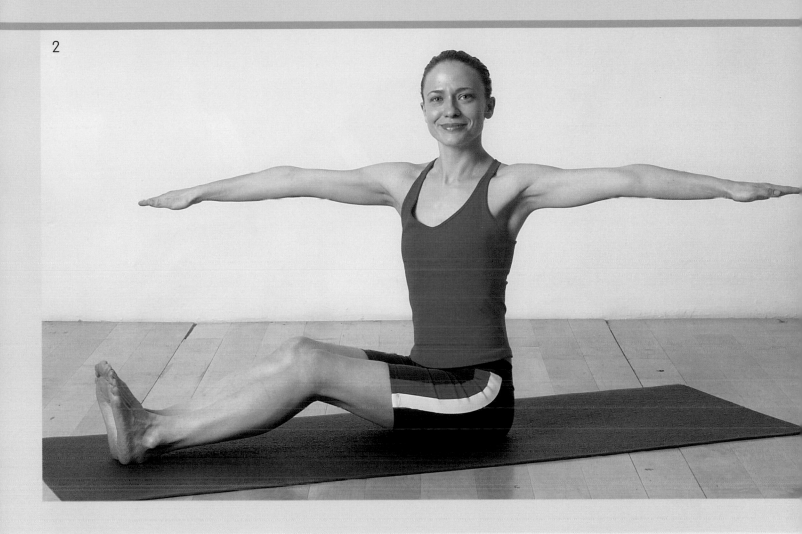

Key Points:

- Lengthen your head to the ceiling.

- Keep your shoulder blades pulling down your back.

- Extend through the heels.

- Twist from the waistline, not the hips.

- Do not let the shoulders raise up or allow the back to round as you twist. You need a certain amount of flexibility to sit up in this position.

- Do not let the feet move.

Progression from:

Beginner's Twist, page 44.

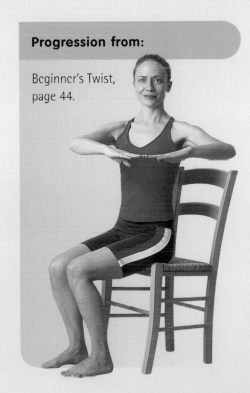

Challenge:

Spine Twist, page 197.

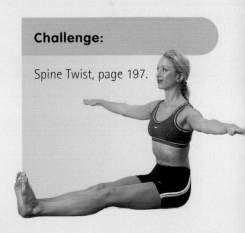

Triceps Push-ups

This exercise is included to give a solid base for the Push-ups in the next section, as they are often performed incorrectly. Perform the movements slowly and accurately, keeping the back long while strengthening the backs of the arms and the abdominals.

1 Lie on your stomach with your knees bent and your hands underneath your shoulders. Glue your elbows into your ribs pointing towards the ceiling. Squeeze your buttocks and pull your navel into your spine.

2 Exhale and press your body straight up, keeping your shoulders, knees and hips all in line. Keep your elbows glued into your ribs while extending them. Your neck and head should be in line with your spine and your focus should be at a slight diagonal down.

3 Inhale as you lower yourself down letting your elbows brush past your ribs.

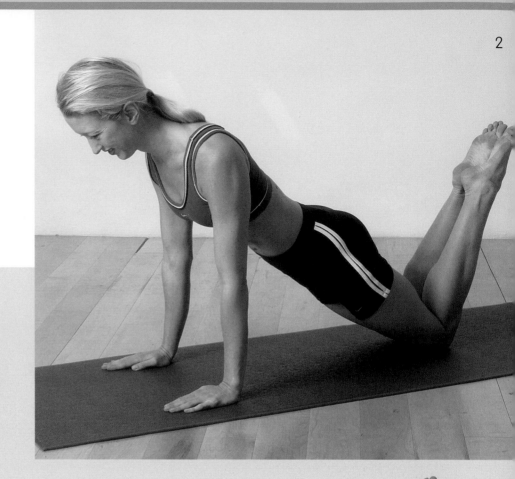

2

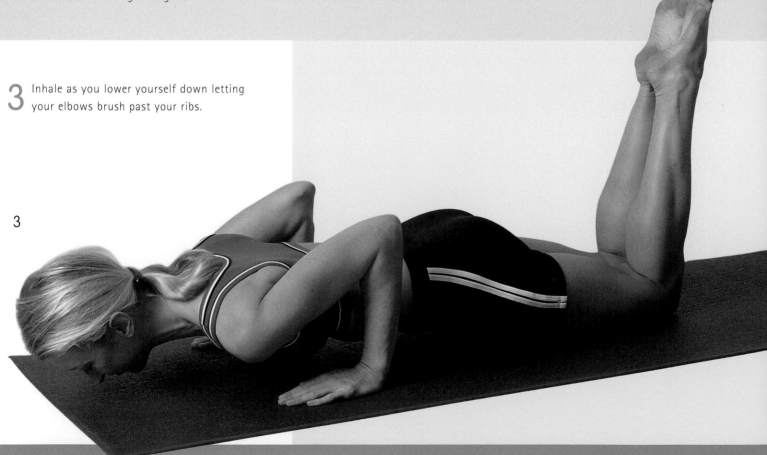

3

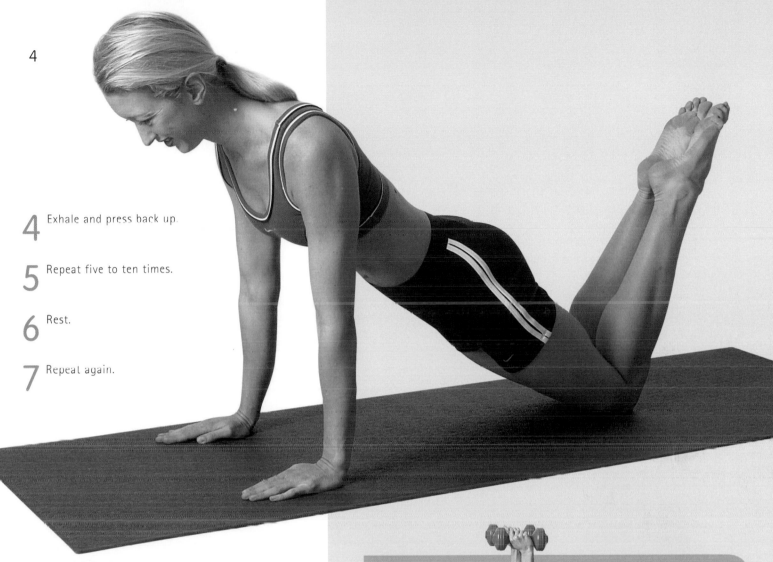

4 Exhale and press back up.

5 Repeat five to ten times.

6 Rest.

7 Repeat again.

Key Points:

- Keep the head, shoulders, hips and knees in one straight line.

- Keep the elbows glued into the ribs.

- Keep the navel pulling into the spine and breathe through the sides and back of the ribs.

- Squeeze the buttocks and inner thighs together.

- Lengthen through the top of the head.

- Do not let the head drop forwards.

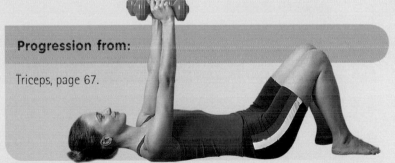

Progression from:

Triceps, page 67.

Challenge: Try the Push-ups on page 240.

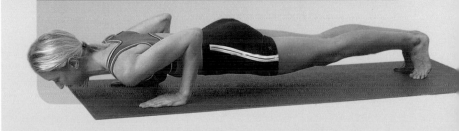

Shoulder & pecs push-ups

This exercise is slightly easier than the Triceps Push-ups because you can recruit more muscle groups to perform the movements. You are not isolating the backs of your arms, so the chest muscles and muscles surrounding the shoulder blades can become more actively involved. Continue to concentrate on keeping the back long and the abdominals engaged.

1 Start on your hands and knees. Hips and knees should be in alignment and hands should be in line with the shoulders, slightly wider than shoulder-width. Weight should be more on your arms than on your legs. Keep the head and neck in line with the spine.

2 As you inhale, bend your elbows and lower your torso down until it is a few inches off the ground. Let your elbows go out to the sides. Think of your shoulder blades pulling back and together.

3 As you exhale, straighten your arms back to your starting position, making sure not to lose your form.

4 Repeat five to ten times.

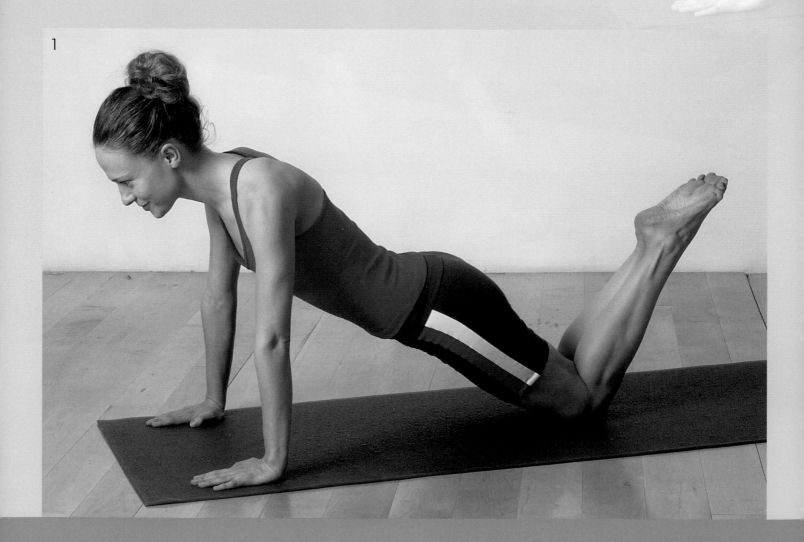

1

2

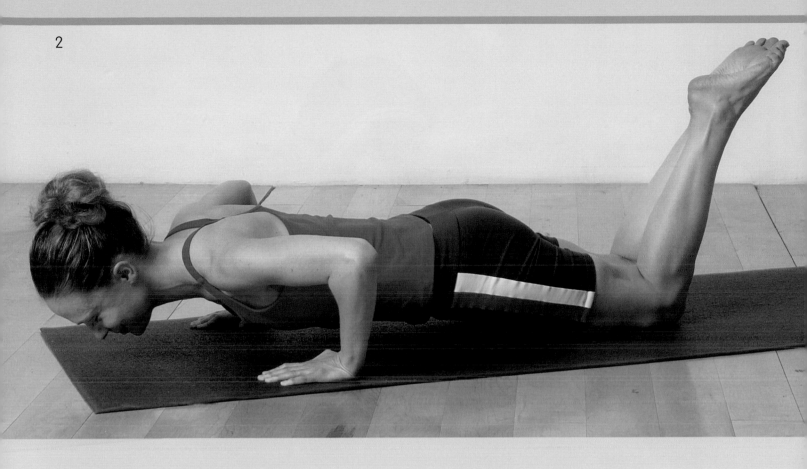

Key Points:

- Keep the head, shoulders, hips and knees in one straight line.

- Think of cracking a walnut with your shoulder blades.

- Keep the navel pulling into the spine and breathe through the sides and back of the ribs.

- Squeeze the buttocks and inner thighs together.

- Lengthen through the top of the head.

- Do not let the head drop forwards.

Challenge: Try the Push-ups on page 240.

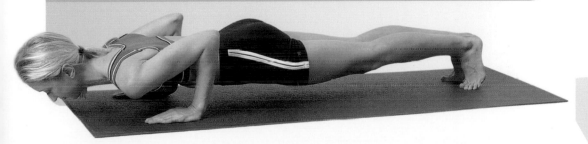

Arabesque

The Arabesque is a great stretch for the hamstrings, calves and shoulders.

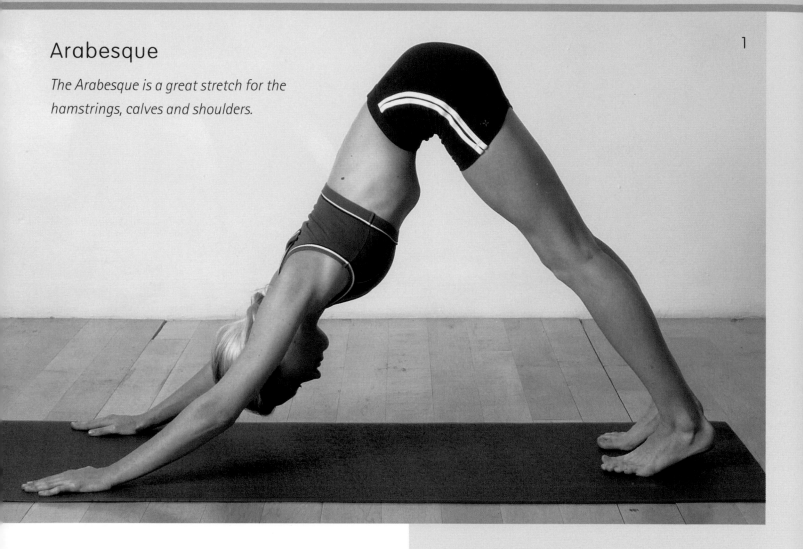

1

1 Start with your body in a high V position. Your hands and feet are on the ground and your buttocks are in the air. Your feet are far enough away from your hands so that the heels will not stay down on the mat. The feet are hip-width apart and the legs are straight. You are trying to press the chest towards the knees. Stay here and inhale.

2 As you exhale, extend the left leg long towards the ceiling, while pressing the right heel down towards the mat.

3 As you inhale, relax the leg straight back to the original position.

4 As you take your second exhale, extend your right leg towards the ceiling.

5 Inhale to relax the leg back.

6 Repeat three times on each leg.

Key Points:

- Keep the hips square while the leg goes back.

- Keep the navel pulling into the spine and breathe through the sides and back of the ribs.

- Keep the legs straight throughout the exercise.

- Think of pressing out through the palms of the hands and extending out through the toes.

- Do not let the ribs pop out.

*This is a *modification* of an **original** *exercise* done on **the reformer***

2

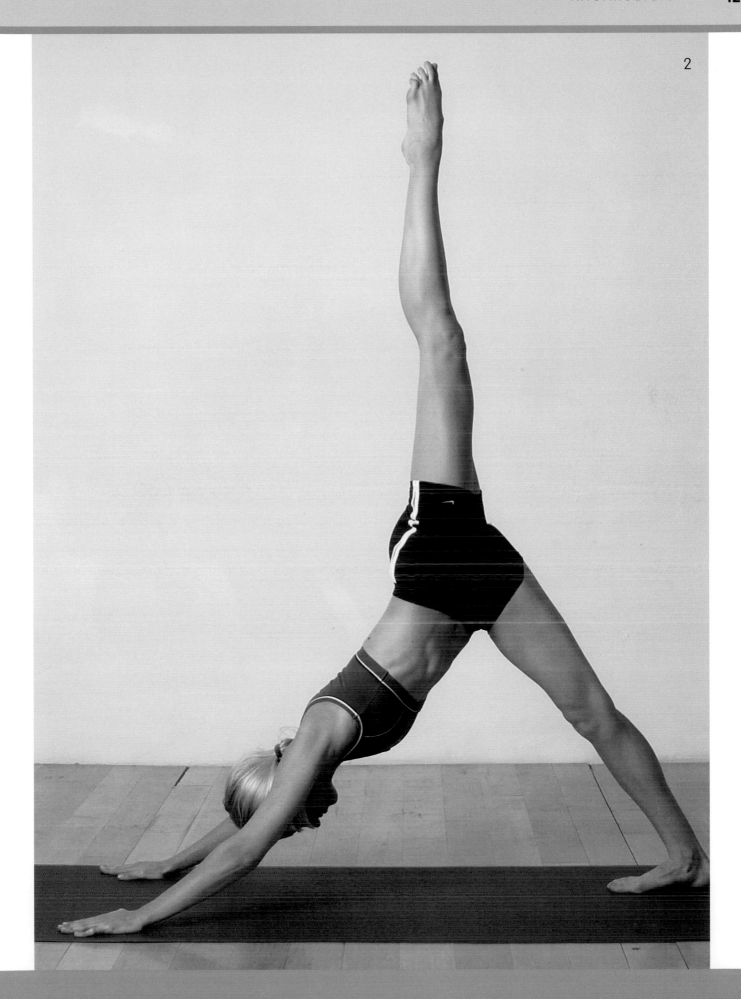

Side Kicks

The Side Kicks are designed to stretch and strengthen the muscles in the leg and hip socket. Think of keeping the upper body still while reaching long out of the hip socket

1

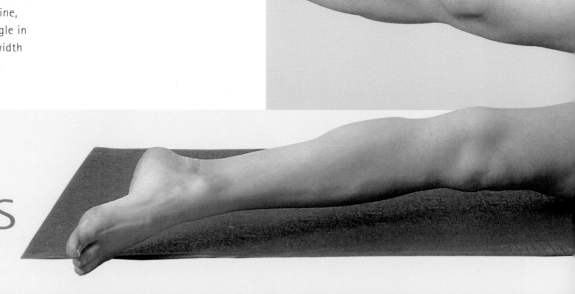

1 Lie on your left side with your head in your hand, right hand pressing into the mat in front of your chest. Make sure your shoulders and hips are in one line, and your legs are at a 45-degree angle in front. Lift up your right leg to hip-width and keep it parallel to the other leg.

*This is an
original
PILATES
exercise*

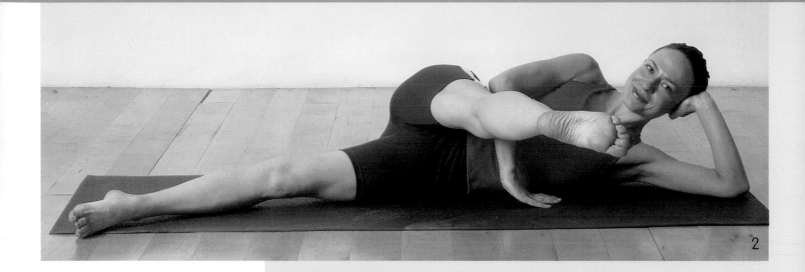

2 Keeping the leg straight, inhale and swing the leg forwards and pulse twice in front.

3 As you exhale, swing the leg to the back and pulse twice. Make sure the torso does not move and the leg stays lifted the whole time.

4 Repeat for a total of ten times.

5 Repeat on the other side.

Key Points:

- Make sure the ribcage and hips stay still as the leg swings forwards and backwards.

- Extend through the toes.

- Keep the leg in parallel.

- Keep the leg stretched long.

- Keep the navel pulling into the spine and breathe through the sides and back of the ribs.

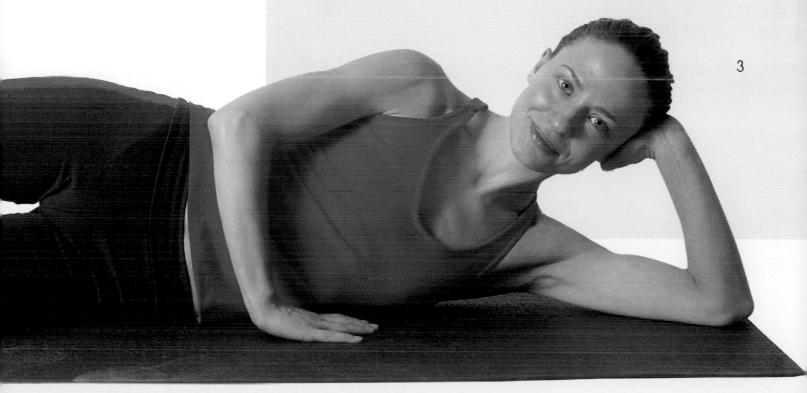

One Leg Teaser

This exercise develops from Teaser with Feet on the Chair in the previous section (see page 69). The One Leg Teaser is designed for balance and co-ordination, as well as strengthening the abdominals.

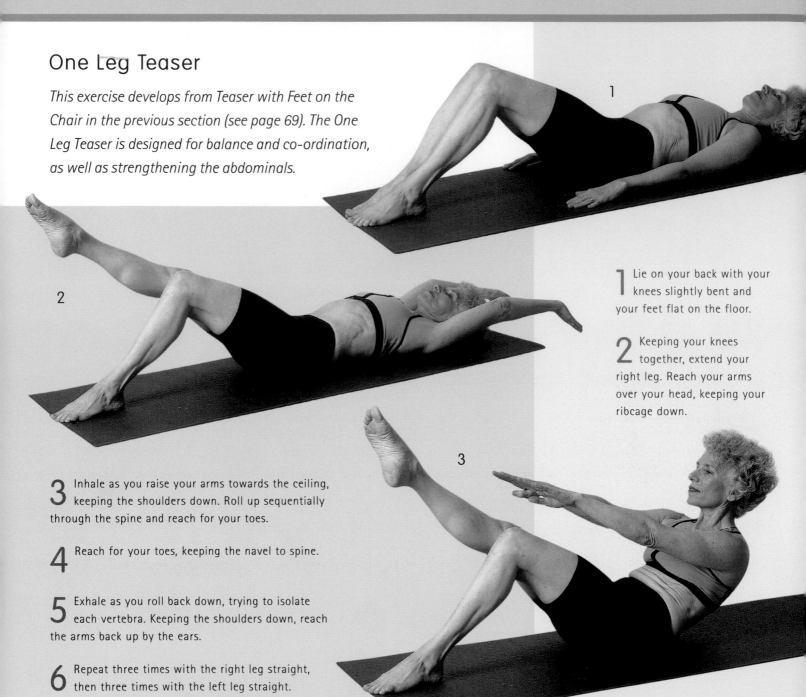

1 Lie on your back with your knees slightly bent and your feet flat on the floor.

2 Keeping your knees together, extend your right leg. Reach your arms over your head, keeping your ribcage down.

3 Inhale as you raise your arms towards the ceiling, keeping the shoulders down. Roll up sequentially through the spine and reach for your toes.

4 Reach for your toes, keeping the navel to spine.

5 Exhale as you roll back down, trying to isolate each vertebra. Keeping the shoulders down, reach the arms back up by the ears.

6 Repeat three times with the right leg straight, then three times with the left leg straight.

Key Points:

- Make sure the hips do not twist.
- Roll sequentially through the spine.
- Make sure you do not arch your back.
- Keep the shoulder blades pulling down the back.
- Keep the navel pulling into the spine and breathe through the sides of the ribs.

*This is an **adaptation** of an **original** PILATES exercise*

4

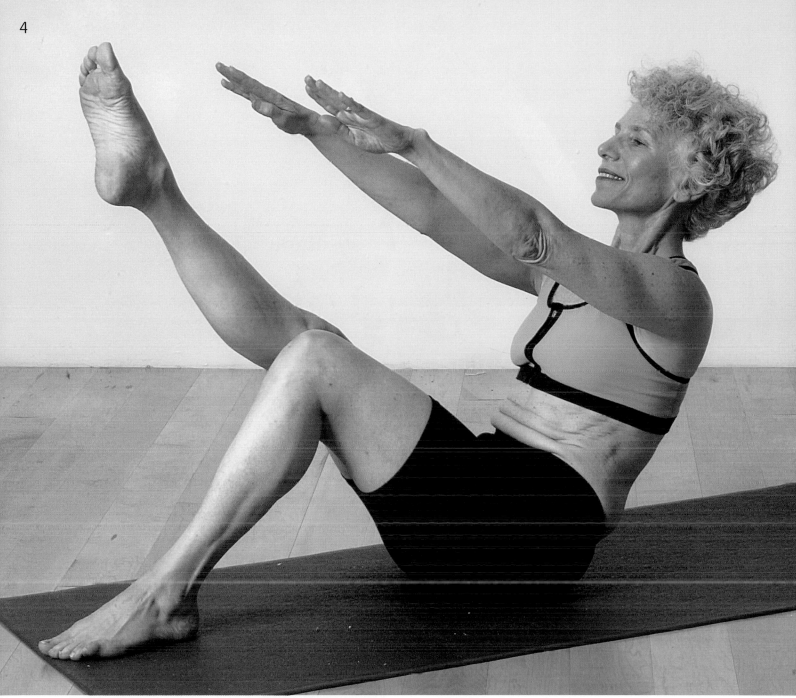

Progression from:

Beginner's Teaser with feet on chair, page 69.

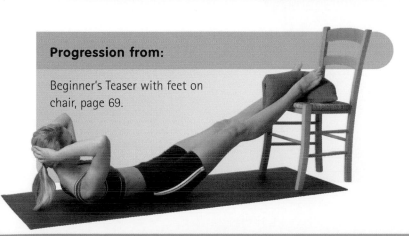

Challenge:

Start the exercise with the knees bent more underneath you, heel closer to your bottom.

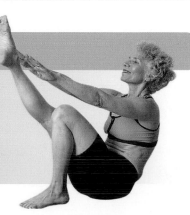

Teaser Knees Bent

This exercise builds on the last one. It is a harder variation because it is necessary to hold your legs up and balance on your pelvis. It also works on co-ordination and strengthening the abdominals.

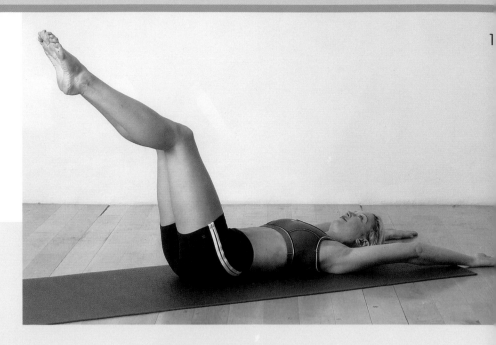

1 Lie on your back with your legs at a 45-degree angle with the knees slightly bent and the toes long. Reach your arms over your head.

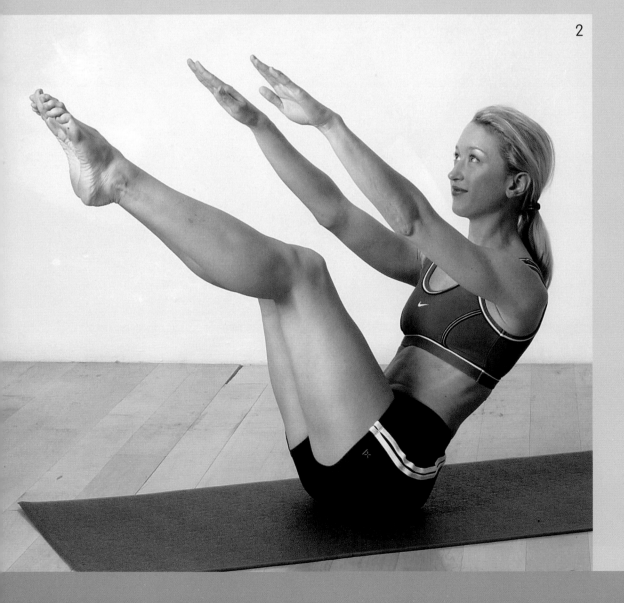

2 As you inhale, pull the shoulder blades down and raise the arms towards the ceiling. Reach towards your toes, slowly rolling up one vertebra at a time.

3 Balance on your pelvis and reach towards your toes.

4 As you exhale, slowly roll backwards one vertebra at a time and pull your shoulder blades down as you reach your arms over your head.

5 Repeat the whole exercise three times.

Key Points:

- Keep the shoulder blades pulling down the back.

- Keep the navel pulling into the spine and breathe through the sides of the ribs.

- Squeeze the inner thighs and buttocks tightly together to support the lower spine.

- Make sure you do not whip the arms.

- Make sure you do not arch your back.

*This is an **adaptation** of an **original** PILATES exercise*

Challenge: Teaser 1, page 210.

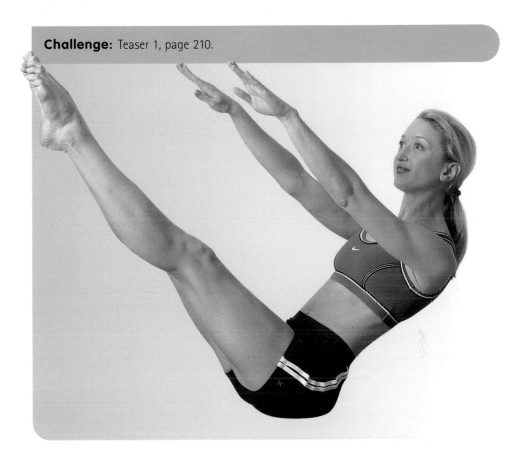

Progression from: One Leg Teaser, page 130.

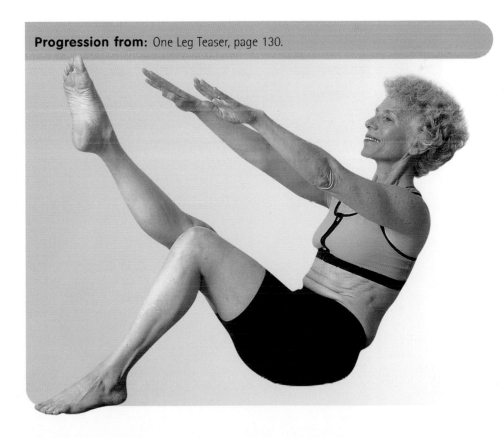

Teaser 2 on Elbows

This exercise is for the lower abdominals.

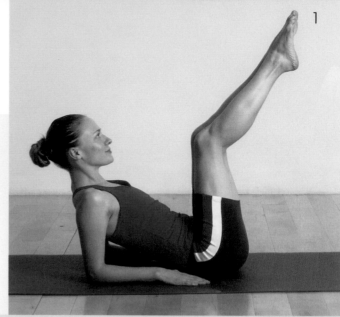

1

1 Start in a sitting position on the mat. Relax backwards on to the elbows, making sure you do not sink into the shoulders. Bend your knees up towards the ceiling.

2 As you inhale, engage your upper abdominals to lower the legs towards the ground only as far as you can control without arching or moving your back.

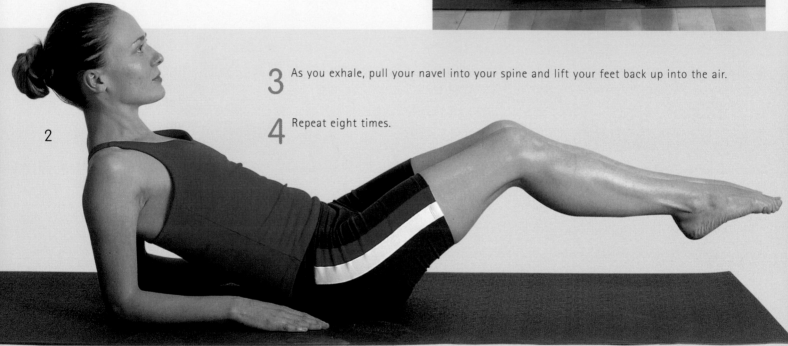

2

3 As you exhale, pull your navel into your spine and lift your feet back up into the air.

4 Repeat eight times.

Key Points:

- Make sure you are lifting up and out of your shoulders.

- Squeeze your buttocks and inner thighs to support the lower back.

- Keep your neck long.

Challenge:

Once you have mastered this exercise, try the Teaser 2 on page 213.

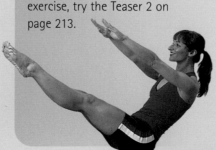

*This is an **adaptation** *of an*
original PILATES
exercise *

Progression from:

Double Bent Leg Stretch, page 104.

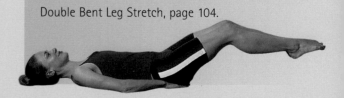

Hug Knees to Chest

This is a wonderful stretch for your lower back and hips. It is especially beneficial at the end of a workout.

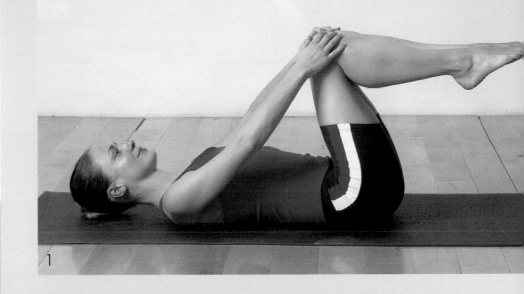

1 Lie on your back and hug your knees into your chest. Hold one hand on top of each knee. Take a breath, inhaling.

2 As you exhale, pull your knees into your chest.

3 Repeat three times.

Key Points:

- Please avoid this exercise if you have knee problems.

- Keep your shoulder blades down your back.

- Keep your neck long.

- Keep your navel pulling into your spine and breathe through the sides and back of your ribs.

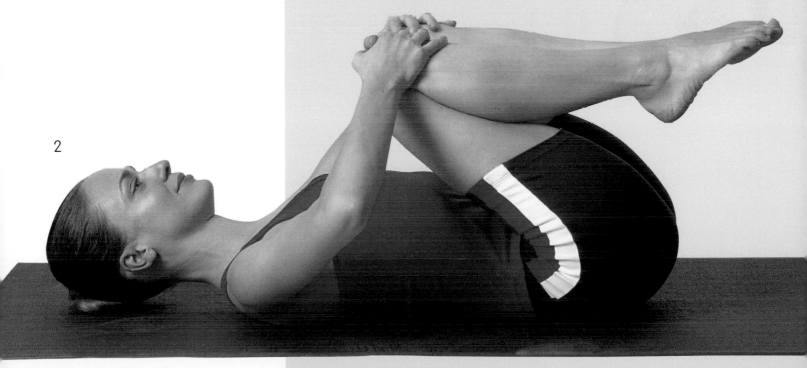

Intermediate 15-minute workout

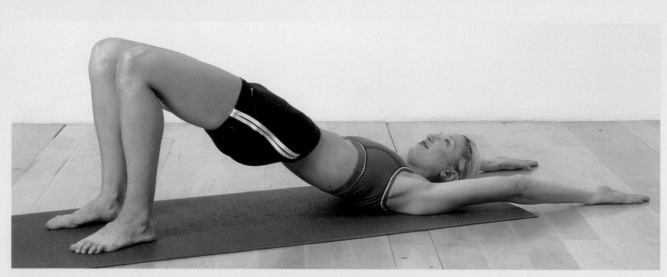

Pelvic Curls with Arms, page 80

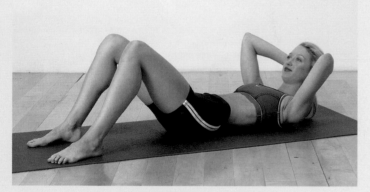

Intermediate Abdominals, page 82

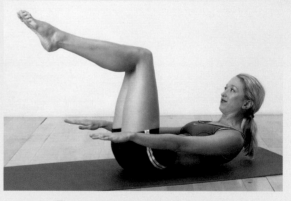

Elementary Hundred, page 90

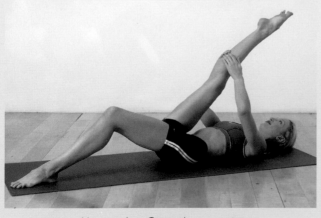

Hamstring Stretch, page 94

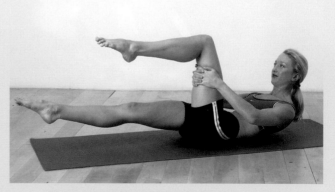

Elementary Single Leg Stretch, page 100

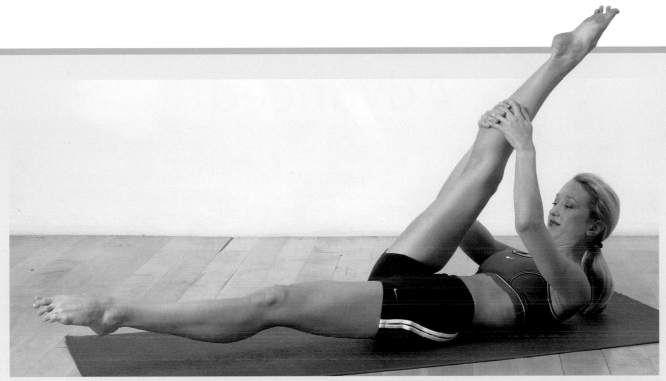

Single Straight Leg Stretch, page 102

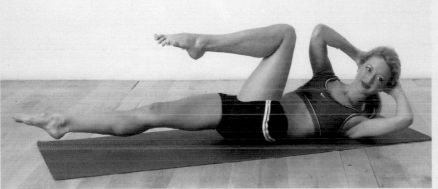

Criss Cross, page 106

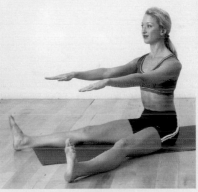

Spine Stretch Forward, 108

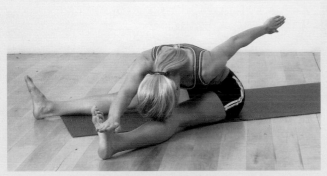

Saw, page 118

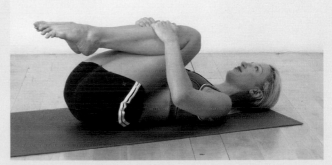

Hug Knees to Chest, page 135

Advanced

'To neglect one's body for any other advantage in life is the greatest of follies.'

Arthur Schopenhauer

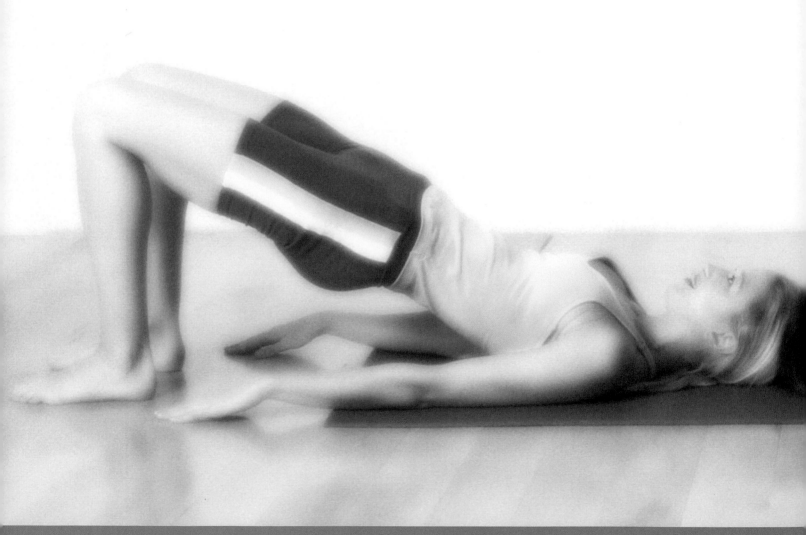

'My back pays tribute to Pilates every day. The response astounds me. I walk tall. I stand straight. I support my disjointed joints with a series of moans and groans. Pilates is the adhesive that holds my mind, body and spirit together. It allows my body to talk to me. I listen. My body thanks me every day.'

Andy Gilbert

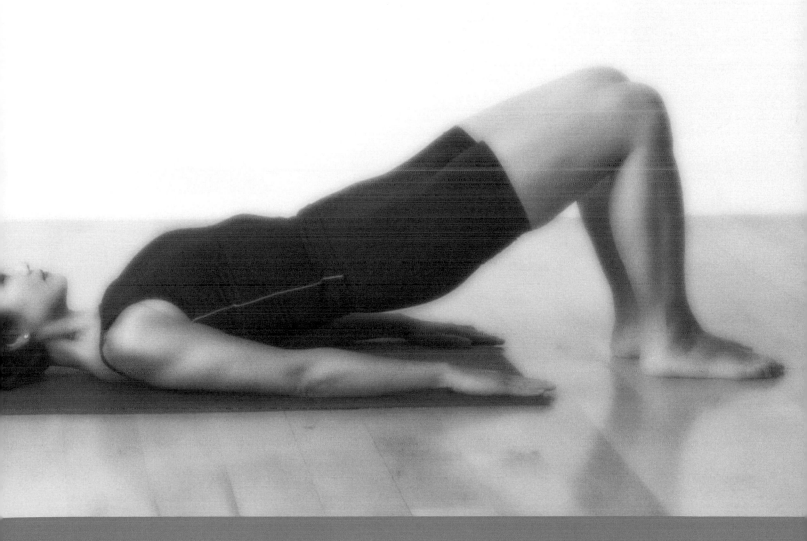

Introduction

The advanced section is the original Pilates Mat as Joseph Pilates taught it. This is the only section that has specific transitions between exercises. Think of the whole routine as a beautifully choreographed dance. Each movement has a specific function and purpose. Focus on all of the isolations you have been working on and transfer those connections into each of these movements.

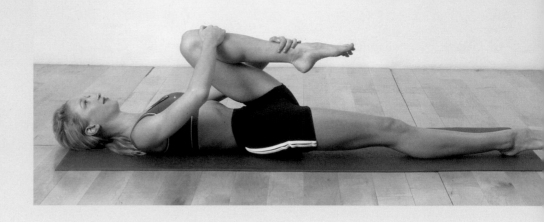

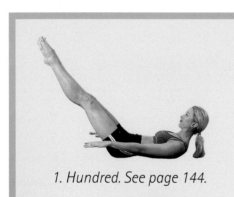

1. Hundred. See page 144.

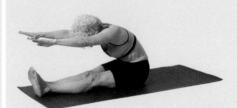

2. Roll-up. See page 146.

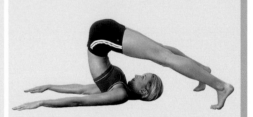

3. Roll-over. See page 148.

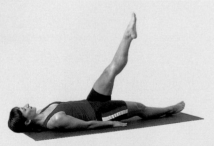

3. Leg Circles. See page 151.

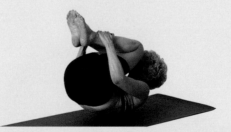

*4. Rolling like a Ball.
See page 154*

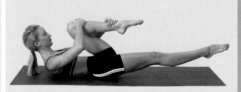

*5. Single Leg Stretch.
See page 156.*

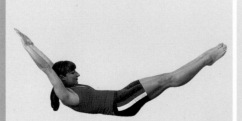

*7. Double Leg Stretch.
See page 158.*

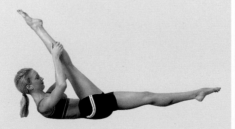

*8. Single Straight Leg Stretch.
See page 160.*

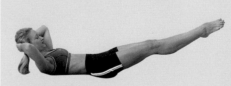

*9. Double Straight Leg Stretch.
See page 162.*

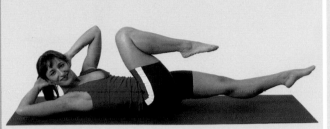

10. Criss Cross. See page 164.

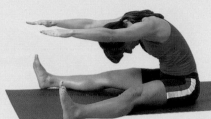

11. Spine Stretch Forward.
See page 166.

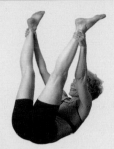

12. Open Leg Rocker.
See page 168.

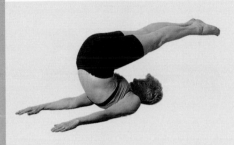

13. Corkscrew. See page 171.

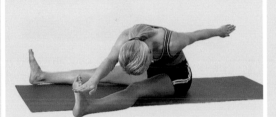

14. Saw. See page 174.

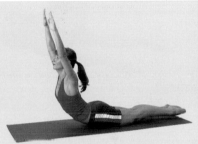

15. Swan Dive. See page 177.

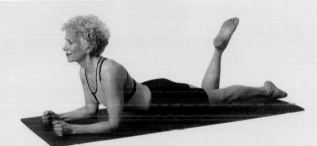

16. Single Leg Kicks. See page 180.

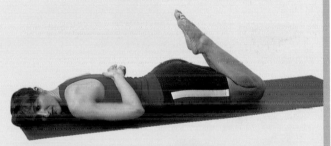

17. Double Leg Kicks. See page 182.

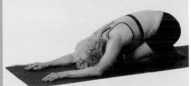

18. Rest Position.
See page 185.

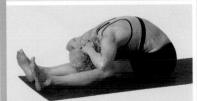

19. Neck Pull. See page 186.

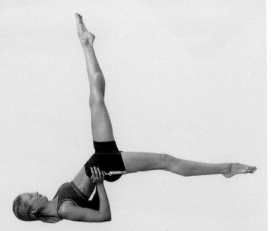

20. Scissors. See page 190.

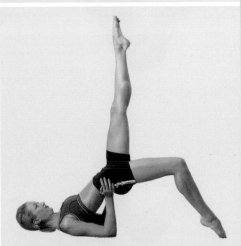

21. Bicycle. See page 192.

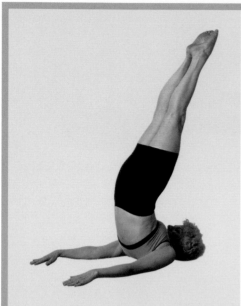

24. *Jackknife. See page 200.*

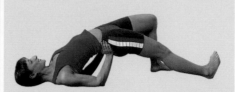

22. *Shoulder Bridge. See page 194.*

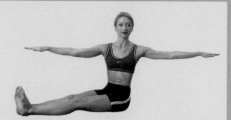

23. *Spine Twist. See page 197.*

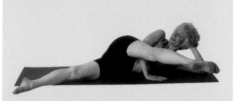

25. *Side Kicks. See page 203.*

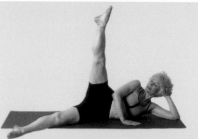

26. *Ronde de Jambe. See page 205.*

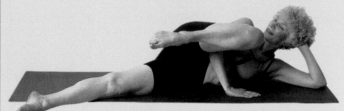

27. *Bicycle. See page 206.*

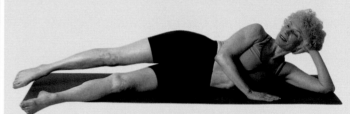

28. *Taps. See page 208.*

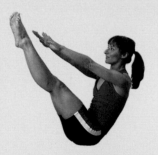

29. *Teaser 1. See page 210.*

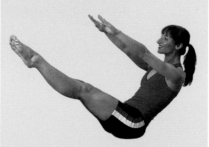

30. *Teaser 2. See page 213.*

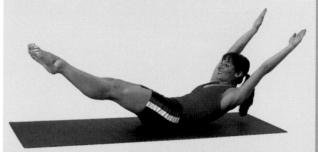

31. *Teaser 3. See page 216.*

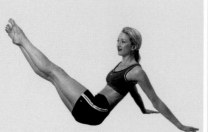

32. *Hip Circles. See page 218.*

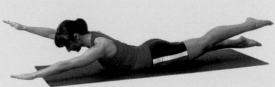

33. *Swimming. See page 220.*

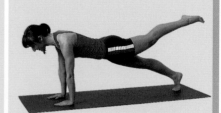

34. *Leg Pull-down. See page 222.*

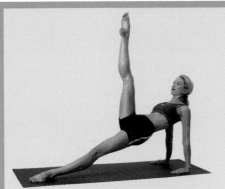

35. Leg Pull-up. See page 224.

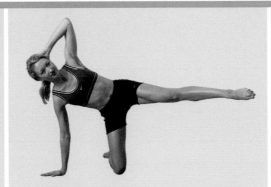

36. Side Kicks Kneeling. See page 226.

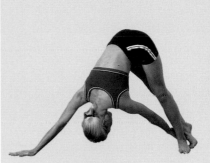

37. Twist. See page 228.

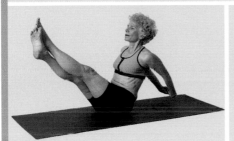

38. Boomerang. See page 230.

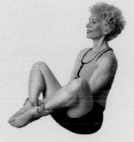

39. Seal. See page 232.

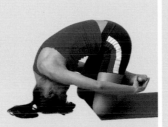

40. Crab. See page 234.

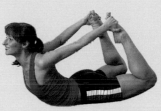

41. Rocking. See page 236.

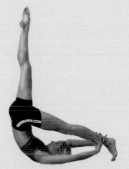

*42. Control Balance.
See page 238.*

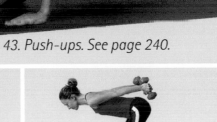

43. Push-ups. See page 240.

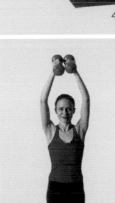

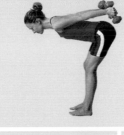

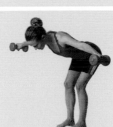

*46. Arms 3.
See page 245*

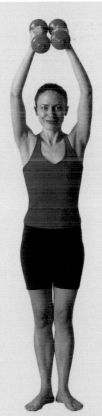

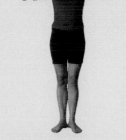

44. Arms 1. See page 243.

*45. Arms 2.
See page 244.*

*47. Arms 4.
See page 247.*

*48. Arms 5.
See page 248.*

*49. Arms 6.
See page 249.*

Hundred

The Hundred warms up the body by getting the blood pumping, increasing circulation and stamina. It strengthens the abdominals, inner thighs and buttocks.

1 Lie on your back with your knees bent into your chest and your arms out long by your side.

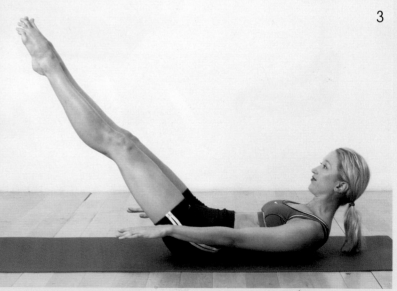

2 Extend your legs up to the ceiling with your toes apart and your heels together. Squeeze your buttocks and inner thighs while lengthening out your toes. Your back should be glued to the mat.

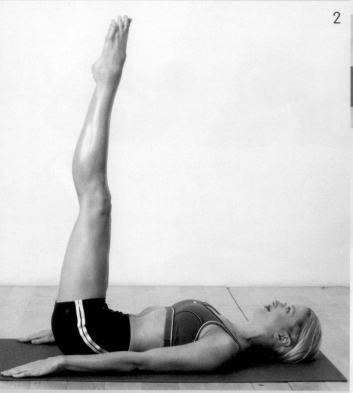

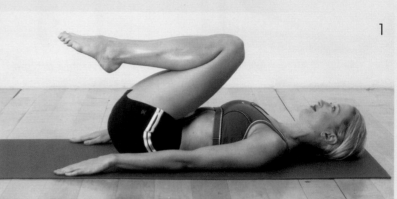

3 Drop legs to 45-degree angle. Pull your shoulder blades down your back as you round forwards from the top of your head. Your chin is into the chest, your palms are down, and you are looking at your navel. Lift your arms so that they are parallel to the ground and straight.

4 Working from the abdominals, pump the arms vigorously 8cm/3in up and down. Inhale through the nose for five pumps and exhale through the mouth for five pumps. Repeat for ten sets.

*This is an
original PILATES
*exercise**

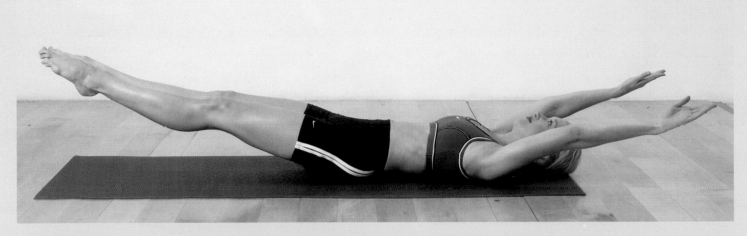

Transition: Slowly lower your legs down straight to the mat and raise your arms over the head keeping the ribs in and the stomach scooped. You are now ready to start the Roll-up.

Key Points:

- Keep your back flat! If you feel your back starting to arch, raise your legs and bend your knees slightly.

- Keep the navel pulling into the spine and breathe through the sides and back of the ribs.

- Keep the shoulder blades down and your neck long.

Challenge:

Lower your legs as low as you can while maintaining a flat back. Ideally, they should be eye-level.

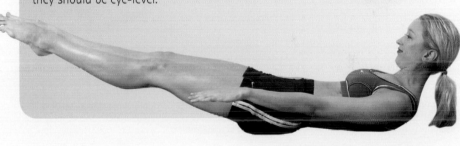

Progression from:

Elementary Hundred, page 90

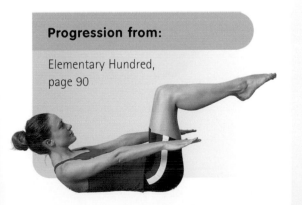

Modification:

If you are finding this exercise difficult, bend your knees slightly in parallel. If the neck gets tired, place the head down but keep going with the movement.

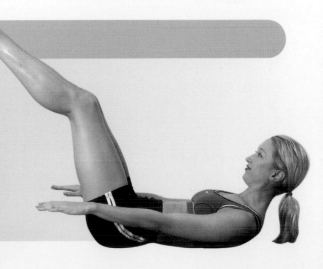

Roll-up

The Roll-up strengthens the abdominals and stretches the lower back and hamstrings. This exercise is ideal for co-ordination, control and flow of movement.

1 Lie on your back with your legs extended straight along the mat and glued tight together, and your arms reaching overhead. Make sure your back is not arching in order to get your hands down on the mat. Flex your feet.

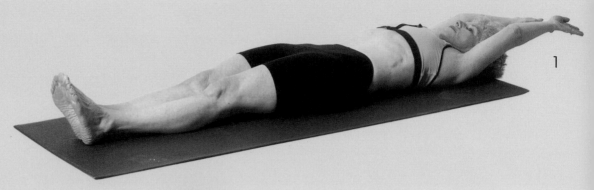

2 Raise your arms to the ceiling keeping your shoulder blades down.

3 Inhale as you lift your head, bringing your chin to your chest, and curl forwards one vertebra at a time. Keeping your stomach scooped and hollowed, exhale and reach your fingers past your toes.

4 Inhale and pinch your buttocks as you roll backwards, vertebra by vertebra. Your hands should remain in line with your eyes at all times. When your head reaches the mat your arms should be extended towards the ceiling. Exhale and reach them up and over to the ground behind you.

5 Repeat three-five times.

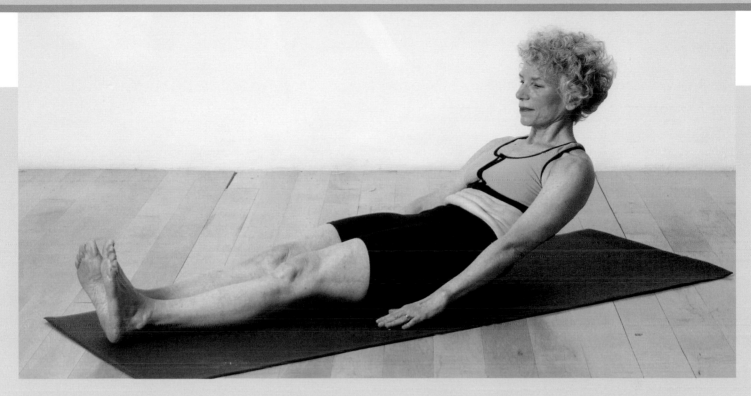

Transition: On the last repetition, keep the arms down by your side as you roll down vertebra by vertebra. You are now ready for the Roll-over.

Key Points:

- Make sure the back rolls up vertebra by vertebra.

- Keep the shoulder blades pulling down the back, and the neck long.

- Keep the navel pulling into the spine and breathe through the sides and back of the ribs.

- Think of extending through the heels as you roll up.

- Scoop the abdominals in and do not let the torso flop on to the legs.

Progression from: Basic Roll up, page 92.

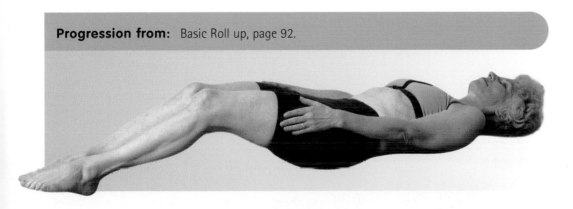

*This is an
original
PILATES
exercise

Roll-over

The Roll-over not only focuses on initiating movement from the powerhouse while stretching out the lower back, hips and hamstrings, but is fun, too!

1 Lie on your back with your legs straight on the floor and your arms down by your sides. Inhale to prepare.

2 As you exhale, pull your navel into your spine. Lift your legs straight off the floor while squeezing your buttocks.

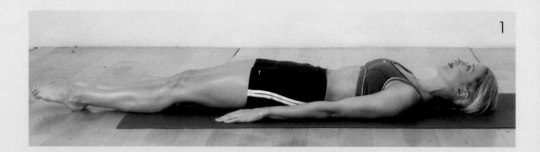

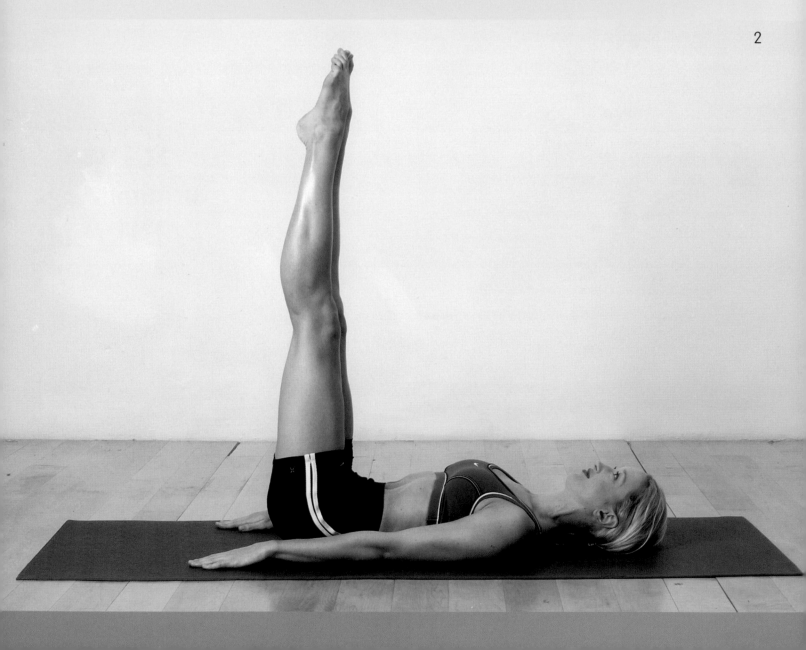

3 Roll sequentially though the spine until the feet touch the mat behind you. Do not put pressure on the neck. Press the hands into the mat and roll on to the shoulders.

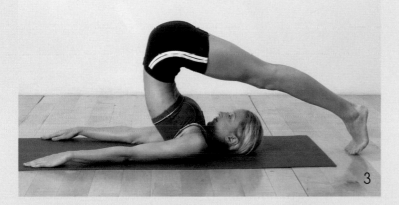

4 As you inhale, open the legs shoulder-width apart.

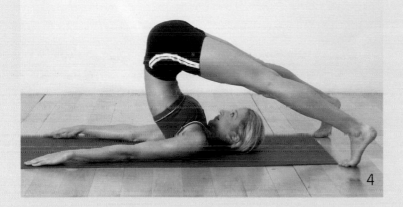

5 As you exhale, roll backwards one vertebra at a time trying to keep the feet in contact with the floor.

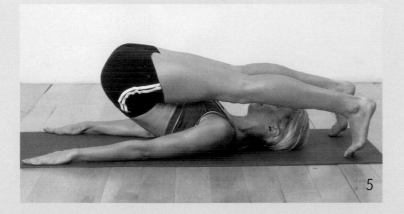

6

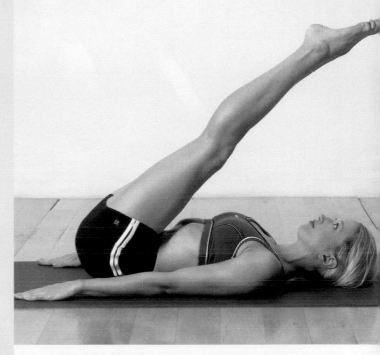

6 As you inhale, lower the legs to a 45-degree angle and close them, keeping the back flat.

7 Repeat three times.

8 **To reverse:** start with the legs at a 45-degree angle. Inhale and open the legs shoulder-width apart.

9 Repeat three times.

10 Inhale as you elongate through the toes and close the legs, zipping them tight together.

11 As you exhale, lengthen the spine as you roll down, vertebra by vertebra. Bring the legs back to a 45-degree angle, keeping the back flat.

12 Repeat three times.

Transition: as you roll down on the last repetition, leave your right leg up to the ceiling and bring your left leg down to the ground for Leg Circles.

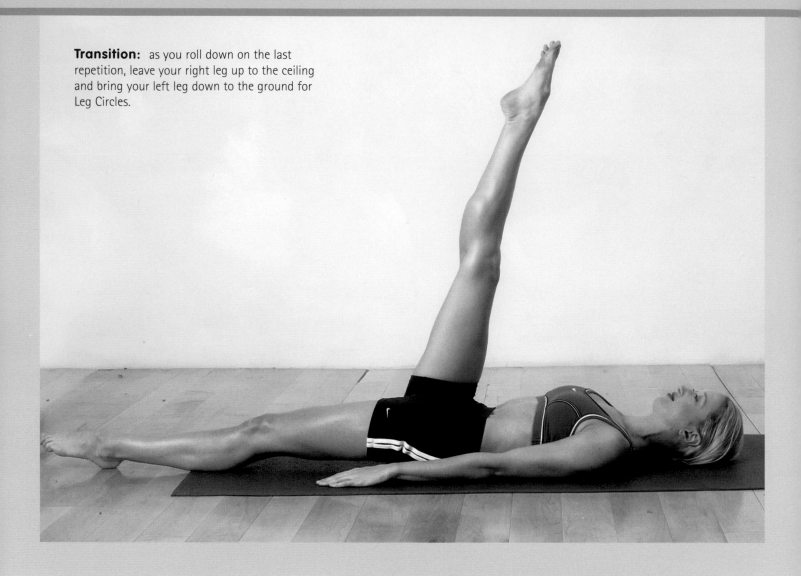

Key Points:

- If you have problems with your back, please leave this exercise out.

- Press the palms flat into the floor.

- Keep the navel pulling into the spine and breathe through the sides and back of the ribs.

- Do not roll on to the neck. Only roll up to the shoulders.

- Glue the legs as close as possible to the upper torso while rolling through the spine.

- Extend through the feet.

Modification:

If it is uncomfortable to touch the ground, keep legs soft and only bring them parallel to the mat behind you.

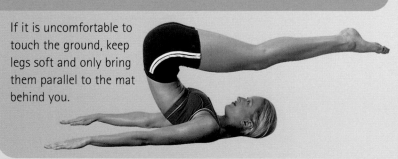

*This is an
original PILATES
*exercise**

Leg Circles

This exercise stretches and strengthens the hip sockets and leg muscles. Concentrate on using the powerhouse to initiate the movement.

1 Lie on your back. Lift your left leg up to the ceiling, keeping your right leg straight and your hips even. Hold on to your left leg and give your left hamstring a small stretch.

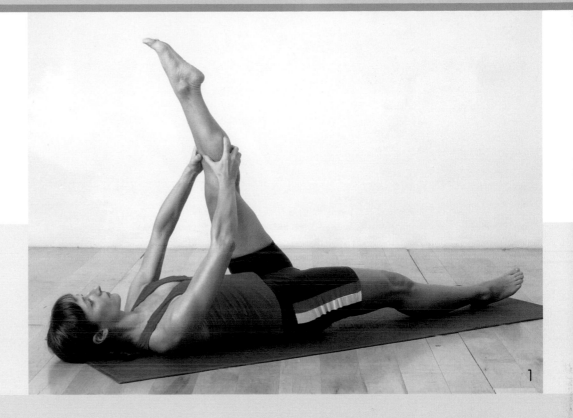

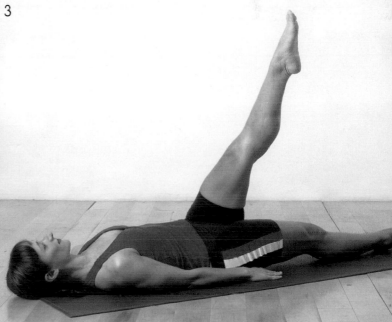

2 Then place your hands back down by your sides.

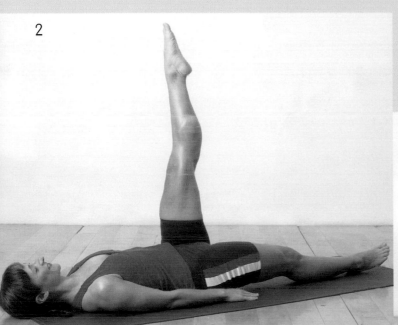

3 Imagine you are drawing circles on the ceiling with your left leg. Inhale through the nose as you cross the leg over the midline of the body.

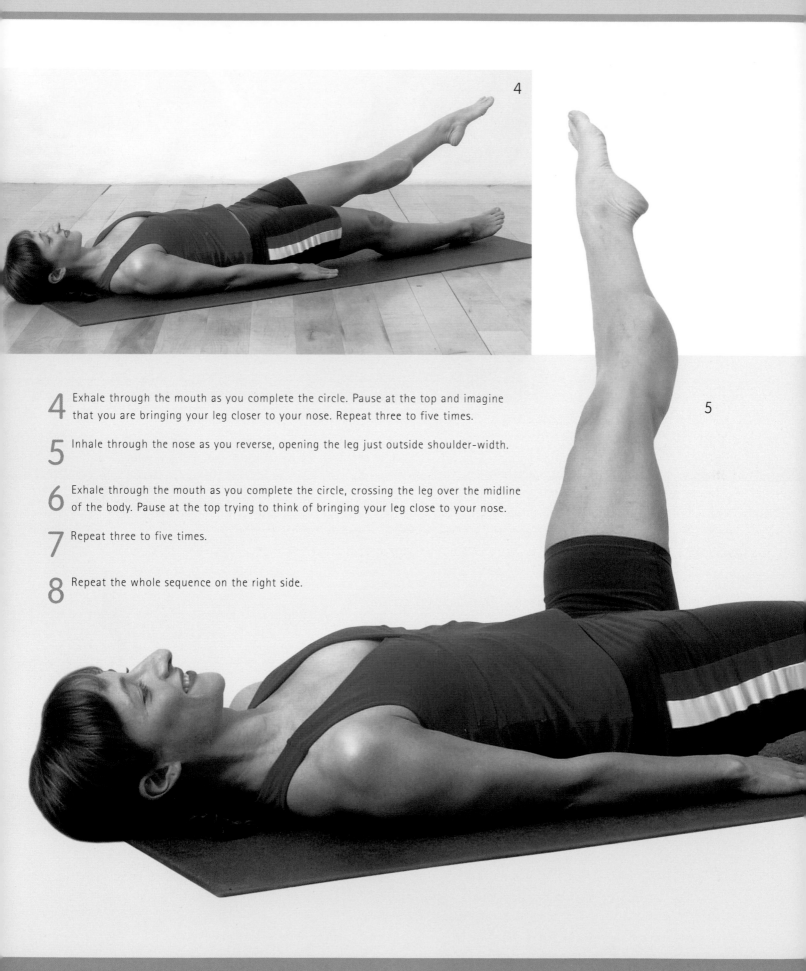

4

4   Exhale through the mouth as you complete the circle. Pause at the top and imagine that you are bringing your leg closer to your nose. Repeat three to five times.

5   Inhale through the nose as you reverse, opening the leg just outside shoulder-width.

6   Exhale through the mouth as you complete the circle, crossing the leg over the midline of the body. Pause at the top trying to think of bringing your leg close to your nose.

7   Repeat three to five times.

8   Repeat the whole sequence on the right side.

5

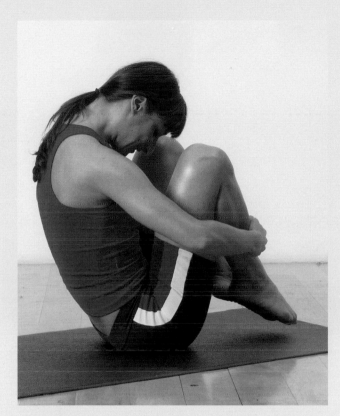

Transition: On the last repetition, keep the arms down by your side as you roll up vertebra by vertebra. You are now ready for the Roll Like a Ball.

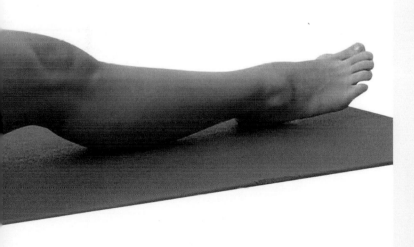

*This is an
original PILATES
exercise*

Key Points:

- Make sure the hips do not move while the leg is circling.

- Keep the shoulders and chest open and relaxed.

- Press the palms into the floor for stabilization.

- Keep the neck long and the chin down.

- Concentrate on pulling the navel into the spine and lengthening the circling leg towards the ceiling.

Progression from:

Basic Leg Circles,
page 96

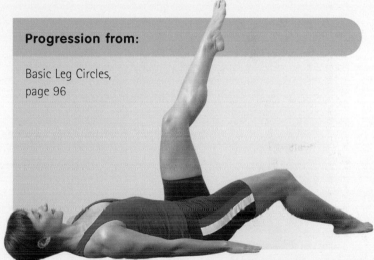

Challenge:

After you have mastered this exercise, try raising the bottom leg 5cm/2in off the mat. Keep the bottom leg still in space while circling the top leg.

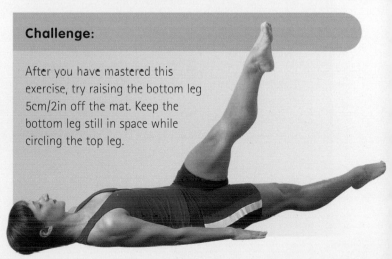

Rolling Like a Ball

This exercise works on mobilizing and stretching your spine and back while strengthening your abdominals. Movement should be initiated from the powerhouse, pulling the navel into the spine.

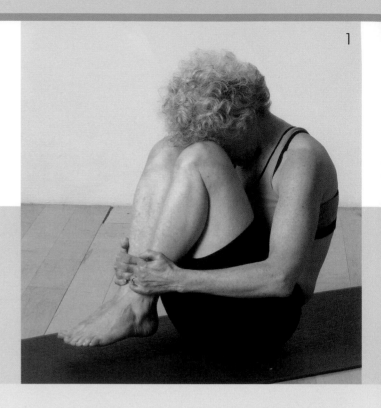

1 Sit up with your knees bent, shoulder-width apart. Your ankles should be together with one hand placed on each ankle. Tuck your head between your knees like a vice. Lift your feet off the mat so that you are balancing on your pelvis.

3 Exhale pulling your navel into your spine as you roll back up on to your pelvis without letting your feet touch the ground.

4 Repeat five times, making sure the position does not change.

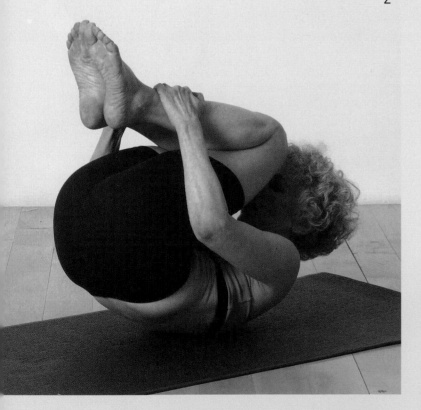

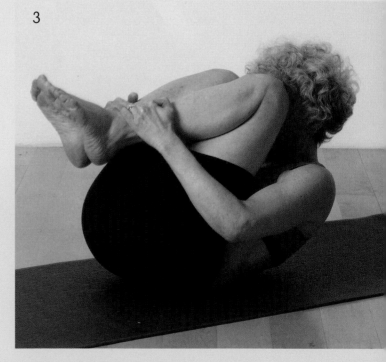

2 Inhale as you roll backwards evenly on to your shoulders.

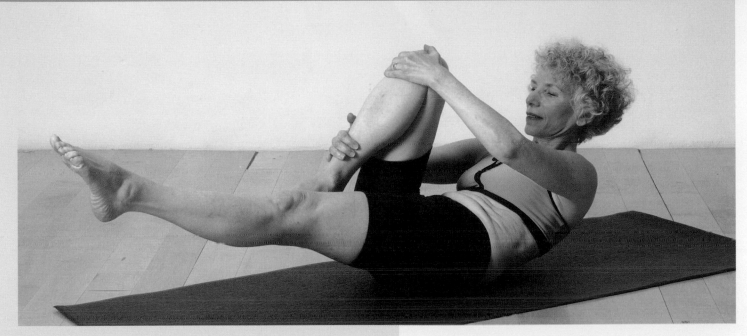

Transition: after you have done your last repetition, place your left hand on your right knee, and your right hand on your right ankle. Roll smoothly down to your back as you extend your left leg to a 45-degree angle. Keep your chin into your chest as you prepare for Single Leg Stretch.

Modification:

Roll halfway down, and then come back up.

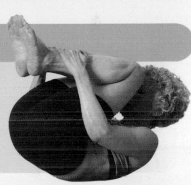

Key Points:

- Make sure the head stays between the knees and the feet stay into the buttocks.

- Make sure you are rolling sequentially through the spine and not going on to the neck.

- Keep the navel pulling into the spine and breathe through the sides and back of the ribs.

- Do not let the chin come out as you roll backwards.

Challenge:

Bring the hands 5cm/2in away from the legs. Roll slowly!

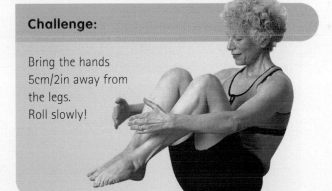

Progression from:

Intermediate Rolling Like a Ball Open, page 98.

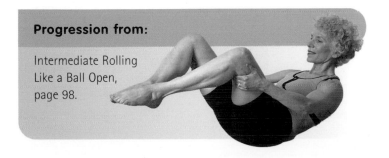

*This is an
original PILATES
*exercise**

Single Leg Stretch

The Single Leg Stretch is the first exercise in the abdominal series. This and the following four exercises focus on the powerhouse by strengthening the core stability muscles of your stomach, pelvic floor, lower back and buttocks.

1 Lift your left knee into the chest. Place your right hand on your left knee and your left hand on your left ankle. This keeps your leg parallel and in alignment.

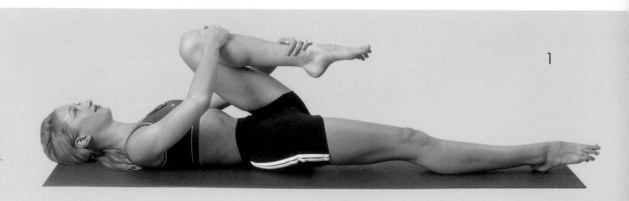

1

2

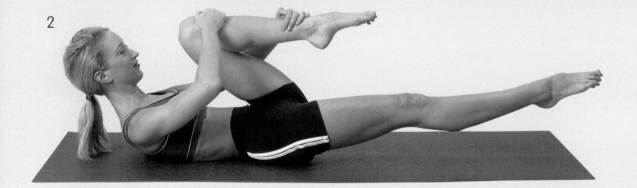

2 Lengthen the right leg off the mat at a 45-degree angle. Pull the shoulder blades down as you curl the chin forwards into the chest.

3 Change legs, keeping the torso still. This time place the left hand on the right knee and the right hand on the right ankle.

4 Inhale for the right and left leg, and exhale for the right and left leg.

5 Counting the right and left sides as one, repeat the exercise five to ten times.

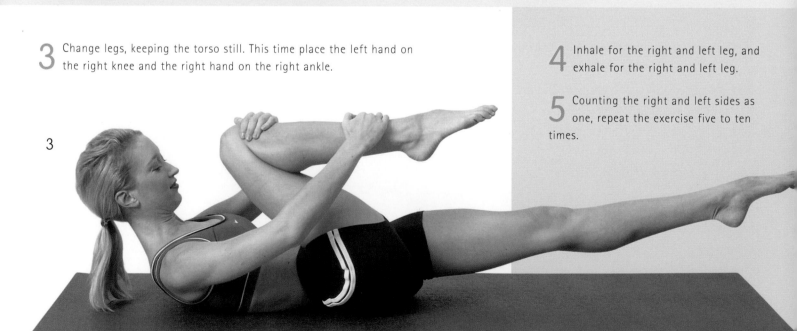

3

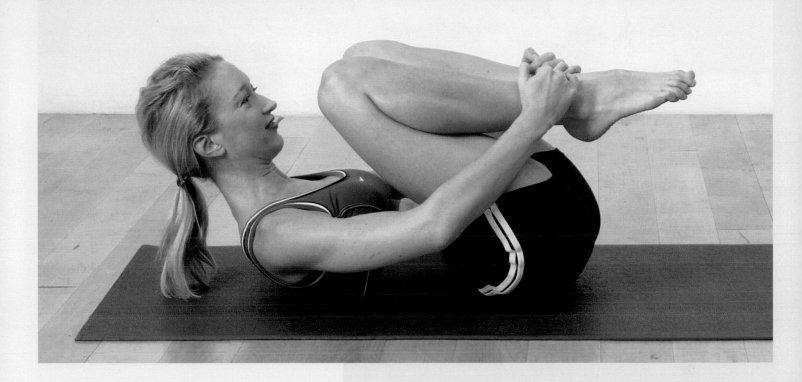

Transition: after the last repetition bend both knees into the chest and place one hand on each ankle. Knees apart, ankles together. Keep the chin into the chest as you prepare for the Double Leg Stretch.

Key Points:

- If the neck is feeling strained, relax the head and keep going with the movement.

- Lift the legs as high as you need to keep the abdominals engaged and the back flat.

- Pull the shoulder blades down the back.

- Keep tension on the arms and pull the elbows out to the sides.

- Lengthen through the toes.

*This is an
original PILATES
exercise *

Challenge:

After you have mastered the exercise, try it with no hands. Bring the hands down to the hips and slightly lift them off the ground. Keep the same scoop in the stomach!

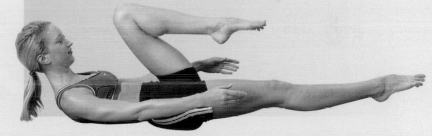

Progression from:

Elementary Single Leg Stretch, page 100.

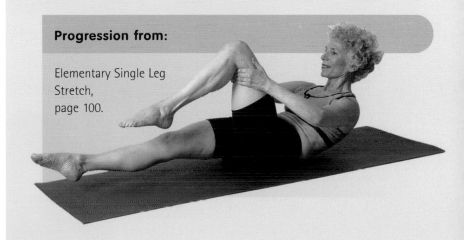

Double Leg Stretch

The Double Leg Stretch is the second exercise in the series of five and isolates outer movement from the powerhouse. Focus on the breath and co-ordination of the movement.

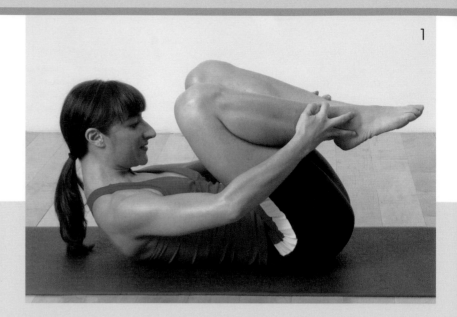

1 Lie on your back with your knees bent into your chest and one hand holding on to each ankle. Curl your head forwards so that you are in a tight ball. Your knees should be shoulder-width apart, ankles together.

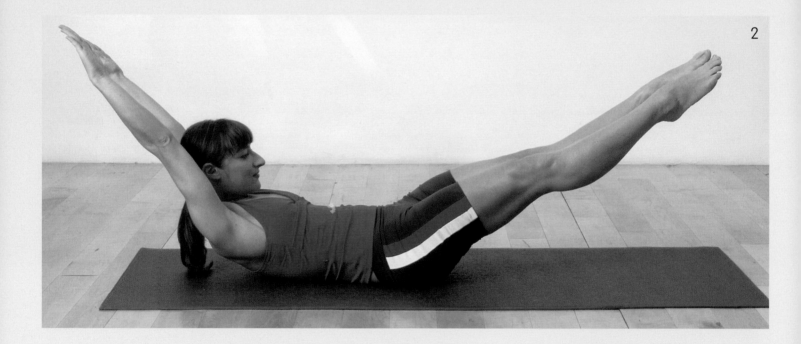

2 Inhale as you stretch your arms and legs out in opposite directions, making sure the abdominals are strong and the back is flat. Your toes should be apart and your heels together.

3 As you exhale, circle the arms around to the sides and hug your knees into your chest.

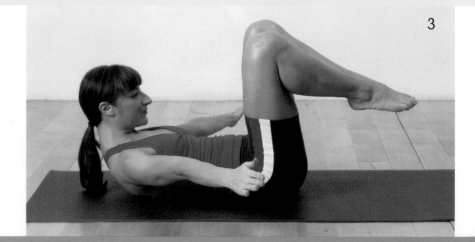

4

4 You should be holding on to your ankles in a tight ball, back in the original position.

5 Repeat five to eight times.

6 Relax your head down and pull your knees into your chest.

7 Turn your head slowly to the right and left to relax your neck.

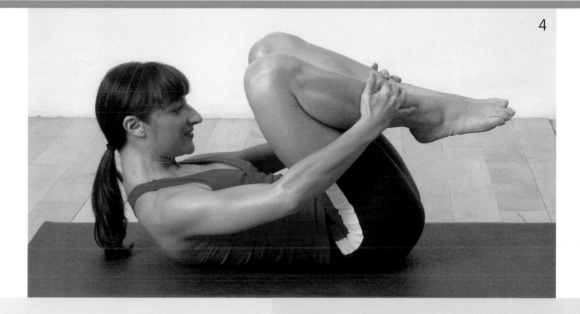

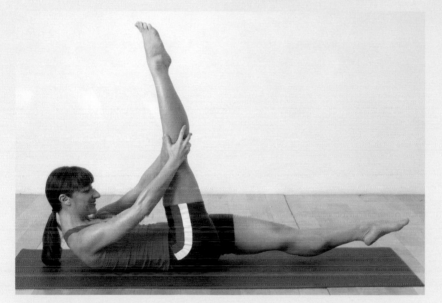

Transition: straighten your right leg towards the ceiling as the left leg extends about 5cm/2in. off the floor. Grasp your right leg with both hands keeping the shoulders down for the Single Straight Leg Stretch.

Key Points:

- If you are feeling pressure on the neck, relax the head down. When you are feeling stronger, lift the head back up.

- Make sure the back stays glued into the mat the whole time.

- Keep the navel pulling into the spine and breathe through the sides and back of the ribs.

- Make smooth circles with the arms. Extend the fingers through space.

- Squeeze the inner thighs and buttocks together. This will help support the lower back.

- Make sure you can see your hands in your peripheral vision at all times.

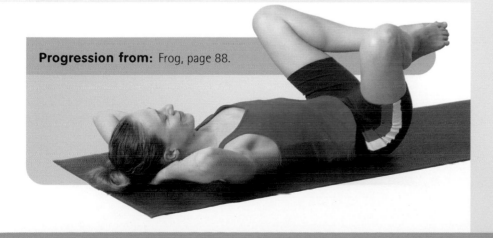

Progression from: Frog, page 88.

*This is an
original
PILATES
*exercise**

Single Straight Leg Stretch

The Single Straight Leg Stretch is the third abdominal exercise and focuses on strengthening the abdominals while stretching the hamstrings. Rhythm and co-ordination are extremely important! Focus on the toes reaching out and brushing the ceiling like a paintbrush.

1 Grasp your right leg with both hands as high up towards your ankle as you can comfortably hold. Extend your left leg 5cm/2in. off the floor. Round the head forwards so that the chin is into the chest and drop your shoulders down your back.

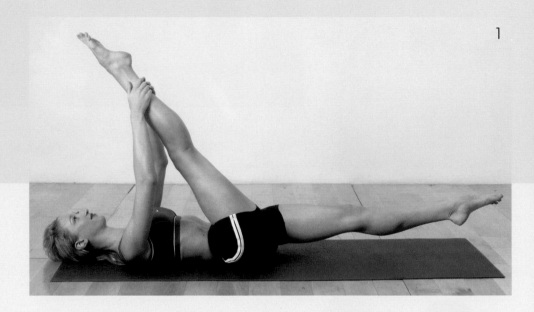

1

2 Pull the straight right leg towards your head and pulse twice.

3 Switch legs keeping them straight.

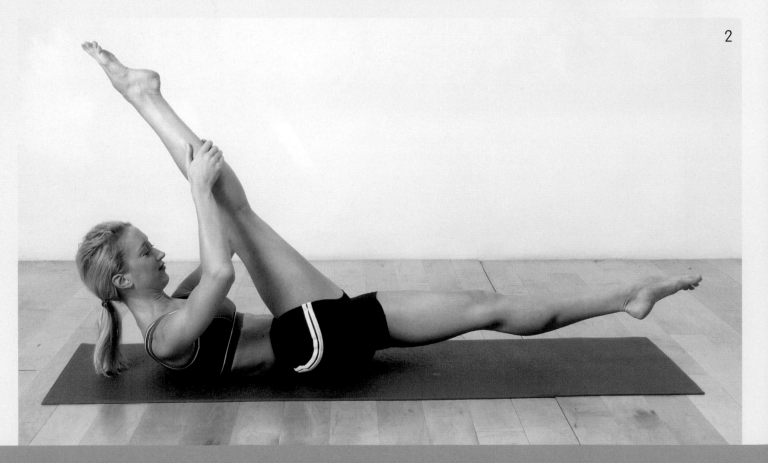

2

3

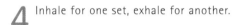

4 Inhale for one set, exhale for another.

5 Repeat five to ten times, counting the right and left leg as one set.

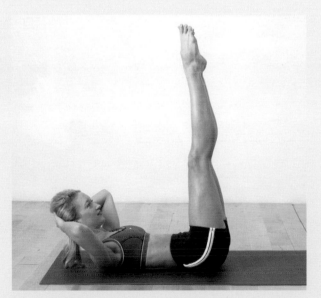

Transition: raise both your legs towards the ceiling with your heels together and the toes apart. Lace your fingers behind your head and round your upper torso forwards so that the chin is into the chest for the Double Straight Leg Stretch.

Key Points:

- If the neck gets tired, place the head down and keep going.
- Keep the legs straight at all times.
- Keep the navel pulling into the spine and breathe through the sides and back of the ribs.
- Keep the shoulder blades pulling down the back.
- Keep the tension on the arms and the elbows pulling out to the sides.

* This is an
original PILATES
exercise *

Challenge:

Bring the hands down by your hips and slightly off the mat. Flex the feet and repeat the exercise.

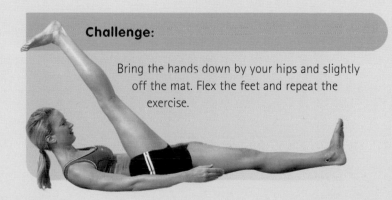

Double Straight Leg Stretch

The Double Straight Leg Stretch is the fourth exercise in the abdominal series and focuses on the abdominals and the flexibility of the lower back and hamstrings.

1 Lie on your back with both of your legs raised to the ceiling with the heels together and the toes apart. Lace your fingers behind your head and round your upper torso forwards, so that the chin is into the chest.

2 Keeping your back glued into the mat, inhale as you lower the legs towards the ground. Only lower the legs as far as you can control them while keeping the back flat.

3 Exhale, pulling the navel into the spine and lifting the legs back to the original position.

4 Repeat five to ten times.

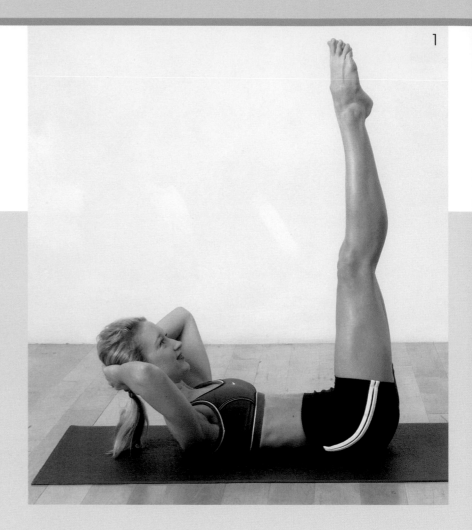

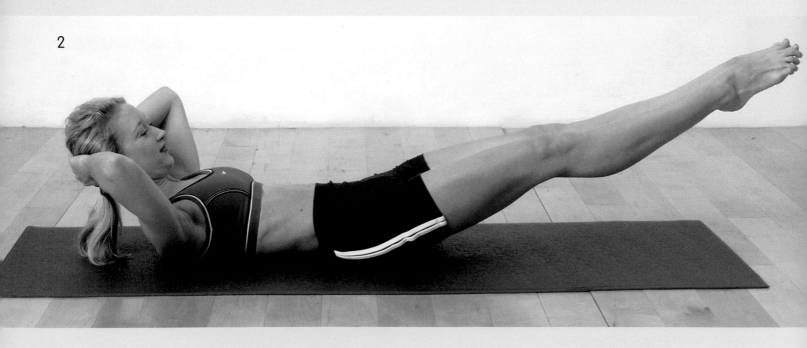

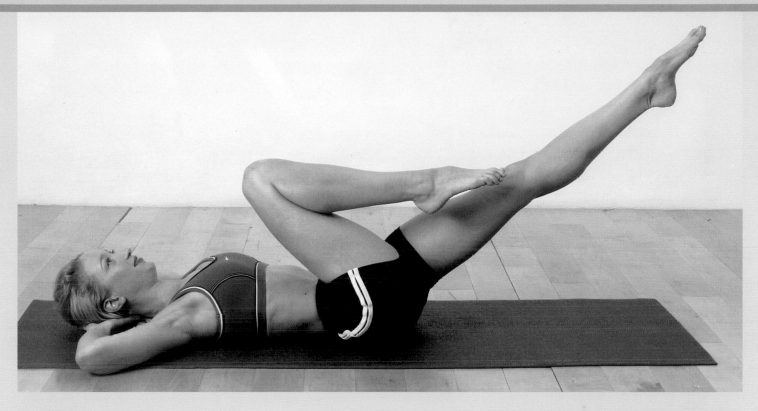

Transition: keeping your fingers laced behind your head, bend your right knee into the chest and extend your left leg at a 45-degree angle in front of you for the Criss Cross.

Key Points·

- Keep your back glued against the mat.

- Squeeze the inner thighs and buttocks to support the lower back. Extend through the toes.

- Keep the navel pulling into the spine and breathe through the sides and back of the ribs.

- Keep the shoulder blades down and the neck long.

- Think of your elbows extending towards the side walls.

*This is an
original PILATES
exercise *

Modification:

If you are finding this exercise difficult, place the hands underneath the buttocks with the palms facing down. Relax the head on to the mat and continue with step 2.

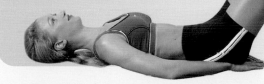

Progression from: Double Bent Leg Stretch, page 104

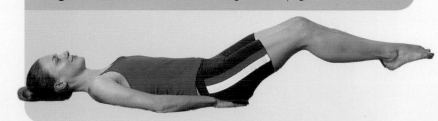

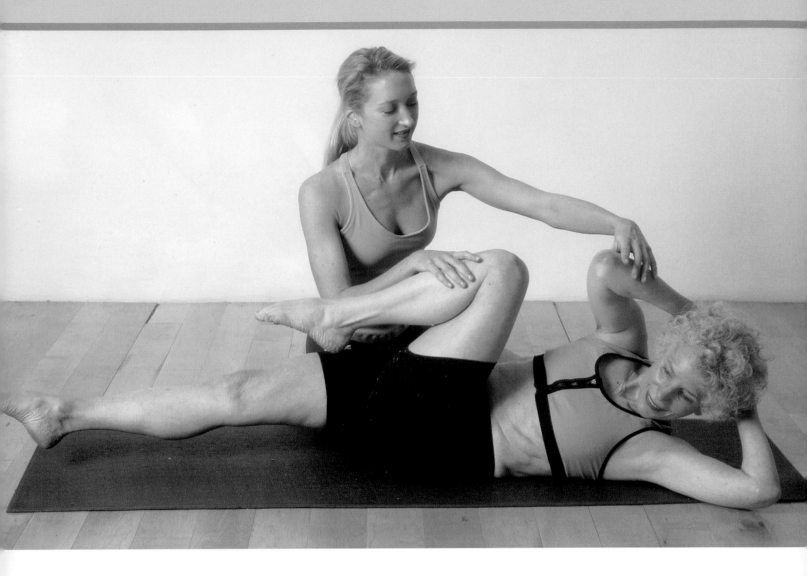

Criss Cross

The Criss Cross is the last exercise in the abdominal series and focuses on co-ordination and control, especially from the obliques. Think of moving fluidly from your powerhouse.

1 Bend your right knee into your chest and lift your left leg at a 45-degree angle off the mat. Lace your fingers behind your head.

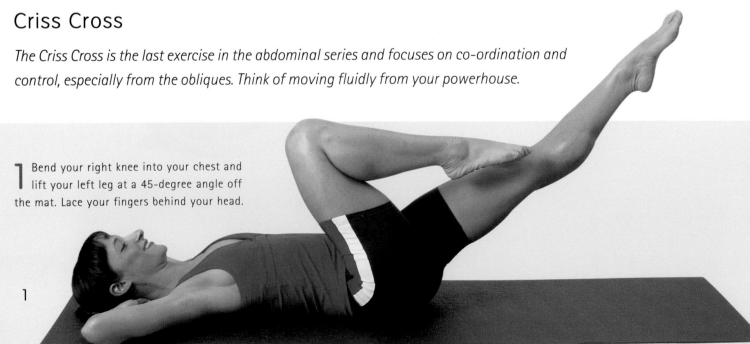

1

2 As you inhale, twist up towards the right so that the left elbow reaches towards the right knee, and lower your left leg as low as you can without arching your back. Hold for three counts.

2

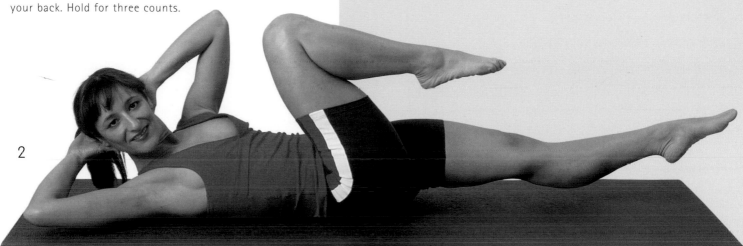

3 Exhale as you twist to the other side, bringing your left knee into the chest and extending your right leg out long.

4 Inhale as you hold for another three counts.

5 Repeat five times, counting the right and left sides as one.

Key Points:

- Make sure everything stays in alignment.
- Do not let the hips move from side to side. Think of the hips being glued into the floor at all times.
- Make sure to straighten the opposite leg every time.
- Twist from the waist and not your arms and shoulders.

*This is an
original PILATES
exercise *

Challenge:

Without worrying about your breath, double-time the whole exercise ten times.

Progression from:

Obliques, page 52.

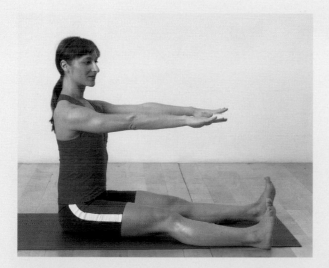

Transition: sit up with your legs straight and a little more than shoulder-width apart, arms straight out in front of you and feet flexed for the Spine Stretch Forward.

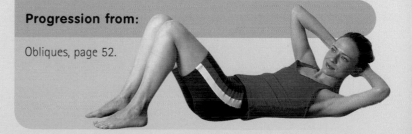

Spine Stretch Forward

The Spine Stretch Forward is great for posture and breathing. It also strengthens the abdominals while stretching the middle and lower back.

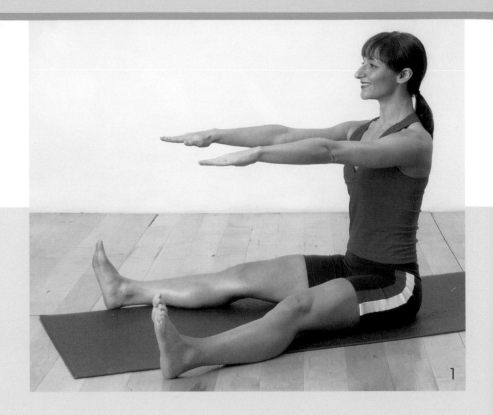

1 Sit up on the mat with your legs out straight just outside of shoulder-width, arms straight out in front of you parallel to the ground, and your feet flexed. Inhale to prepare.

2 As you exhale, start from the top of the head and round forwards, vertebra by vertebra. Think of diving over a large ball in front of you.

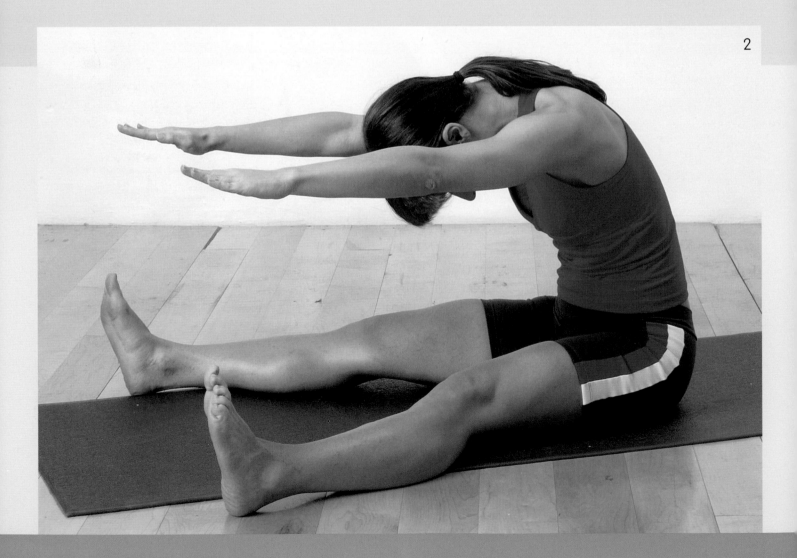

3 Try to keep the stomach engaged and the tailbone down on the mat.

4 Inhale to roll back up to a sitting position.

5 Repeat five times.

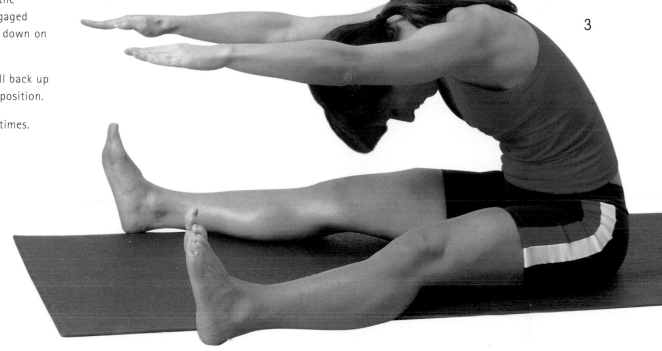

3

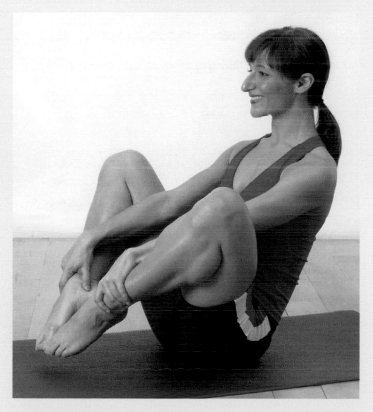

Transition: bend the knees in and hold on to the tops of the ankles with both hands. Lift the feet off the mat and prepare for the Open Leg Rocker.

Key Points:

- While you are sitting up, make sure the back is long and tall and you are not rounding. You might need to sit up on a pillow or bend the knees slightly.

- Keep the shoulder blades pressing down at all times.

- Extend through the heels.

- Keep the navel pulling into the spine and breathe through the sides and back of the ribs.

- Think of pressing the tailbone down and lengthening the head in the opposite direction.

- Keep your knees and toes facing the ceiling and do not let them roll in or out.

*This is an
original PILATES
exercise *

Open Leg Rocker

The Open Leg Rocker takes strength, control and flexibility, but most importantly, it's fun too.

1 Sitting on the floor, bend the knees and hold on to the tops of your ankles. Lift the feet slightly off the floor.

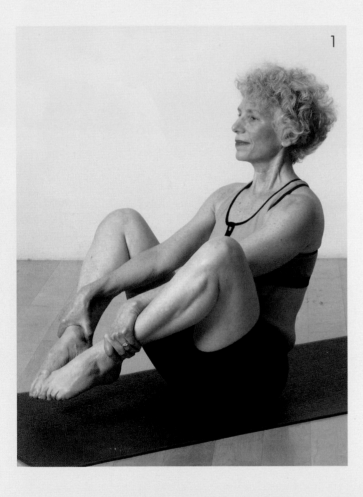

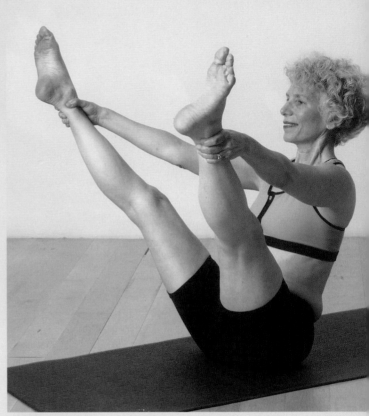

2 Straighten your legs up to the ceiling and spread your legs in a V position just outside shoulder width. Keep your hands on your ankles.

3 Keep your shoulders down and bring your chin forwards into your chest.

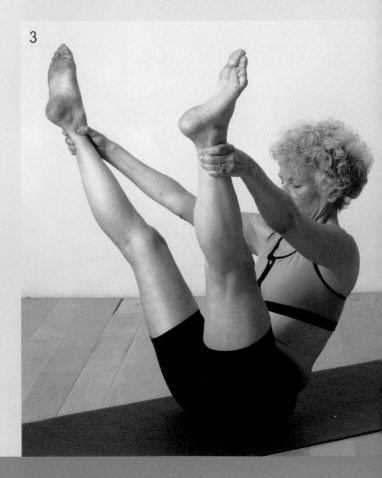

4 Pull your navel into your spine and inhale as you roll your body backwards on to the middle of your shoulder blades. Your feet should not touch the ground behind you.

5 Pull your navel into your spine and exhale to roll back up and balance on the tailbone with your legs in a high V.

6 Repeat five to eight times.

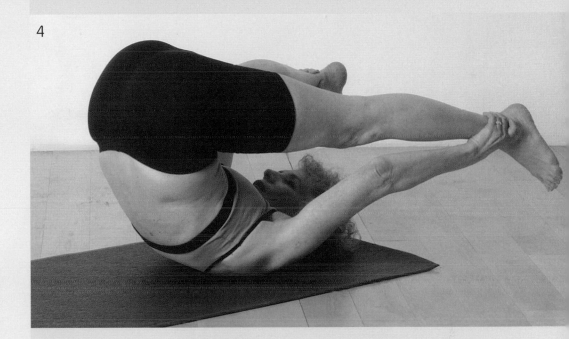

4

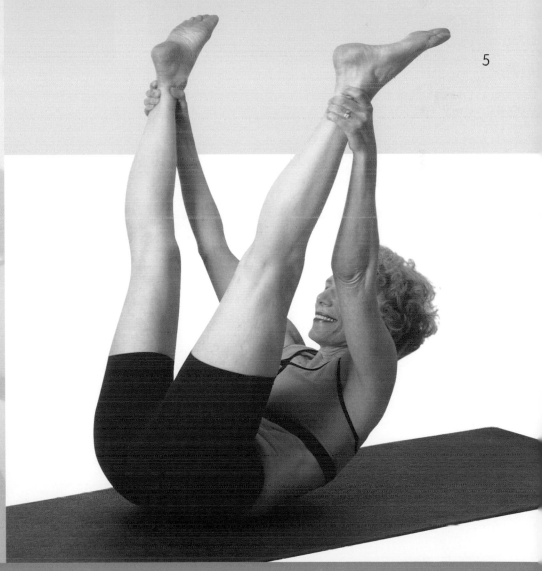

5

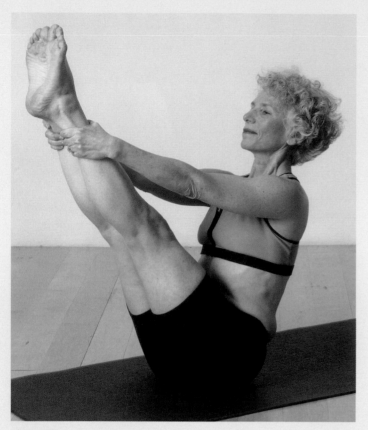

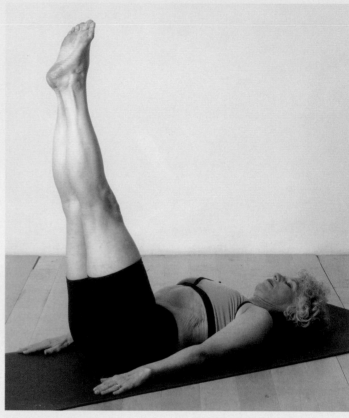

Transition: close your legs and roll down on to the floor with control for the Corkscrew.

Key Points:

- Do not go crashing back on your head!

- Maintain straight arms and legs throughout.

- Do not let the head go backwards as you roll. Keep the chin in.

- Think of the abdominals initiating the movement.

- Do not go on to the neck. Roll backwards onto the shoulders.

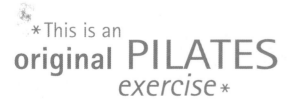

*This is an
original PILATES
exercise *

Challenge:

Once you have mastered the Open Leg Rocker, try holding on to your toes. . .

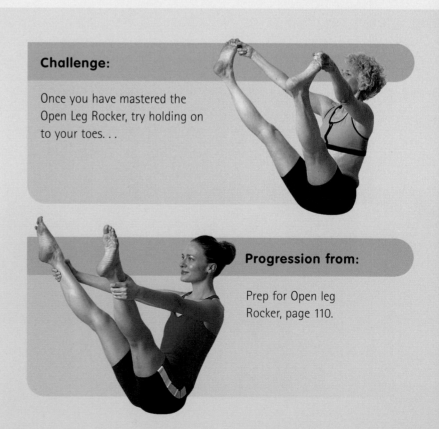

Progression from:

Prep for Open leg Rocker, page 110.

Corkscrew

The Corkscrew is an all-encompassing exercise, based on all the principles of Pilates. It works on concentration, control, co-ordination, centring, precision, flow and breath. This exercise focuses on the abdominals, legs and buttocks.

1 Lie on your back with your arms straight down by your side and your legs extended towards the ceiling.

2 Using your abdominals, squeeze your buttocks and lift your legs straight over your head. You want your weight over your shoulders with your toes apart and your heels together.

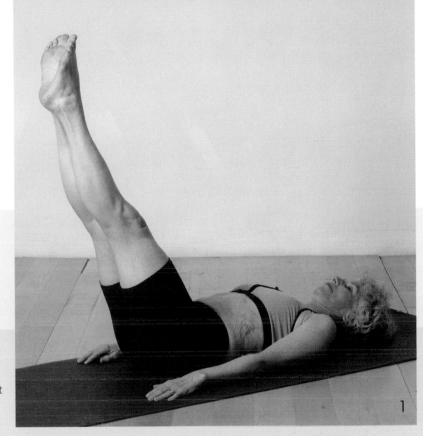

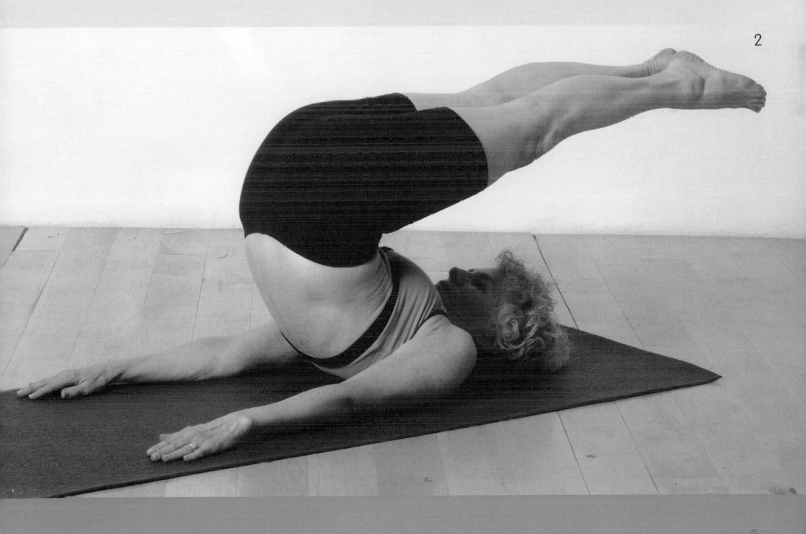

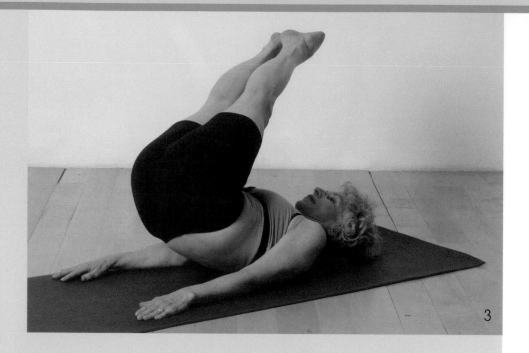

3

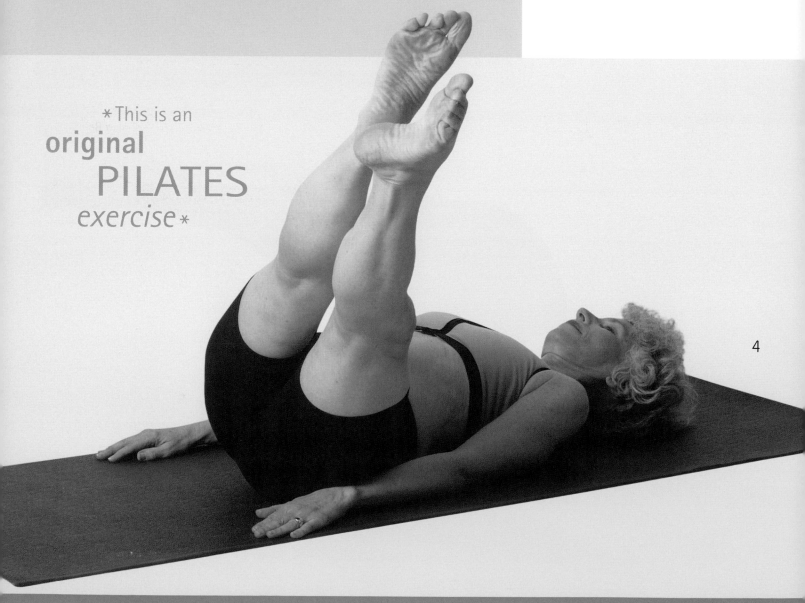

3 As you inhale, lower the hips vertebra by vertebra in a straight line. When your back is flat swing a big circle with the legs on the right hip down around to the left.

4 Squeeze your buttocks and exhale as you lift your pelvis up as the legs go overhead and back to their original position.

5 Immediately reverse, rolling down the spine and then swinging the legs to the left, keep the back flat as they circle down around to the right, and back up.

6 Repeat three times, counting the right and left as one.

*This is an
original
PILATES
*exercise**

4

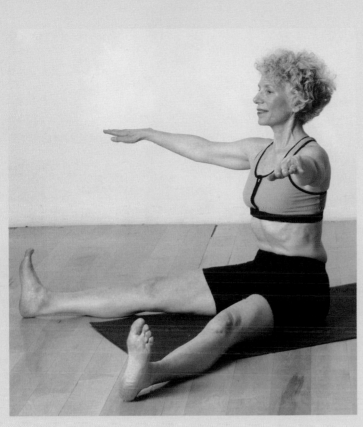

Transition: roll up to a sitting position with the legs just outside shoulder-width and the feet flexed to prepare for the Saw.

Key Points:

- If you have problems with your back, please leave this exercise out. Try instead the Small Corkscrew on page 116.

- Squeeze the buttocks and inner thighs throughout the exercise to help support the lower back.

- Keep pulling the navel into the spine and breathe through the sides and back of the ribs.

- Extend through the toes.

- Keep the shoulder blades down and the neck long.

- Press the palms into the floor for added stability.

- Roll on to the shoulders and not on the neck.

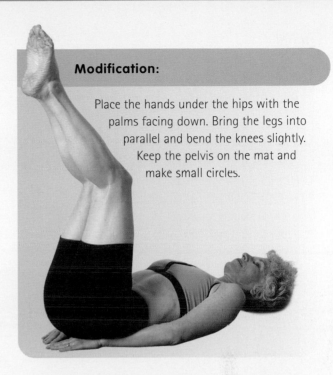

Modification:

Place the hands under the hips with the palms facing down. Bring the legs into parallel and bend the knees slightly. Keep the pelvis on the mat and make small circles.

Challenge:

After you have mastered the Corkscrew, place the hands behind the head with the elbows wide. Repeat.

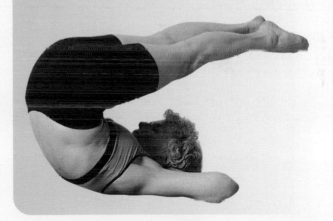

Progression from:

Small Corkscrew, page 116.

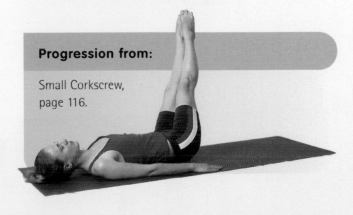

Saw

This is a great exercise to stretch the inner thighs and hamstrings.
It also strengthens the obliques and stretches the back.

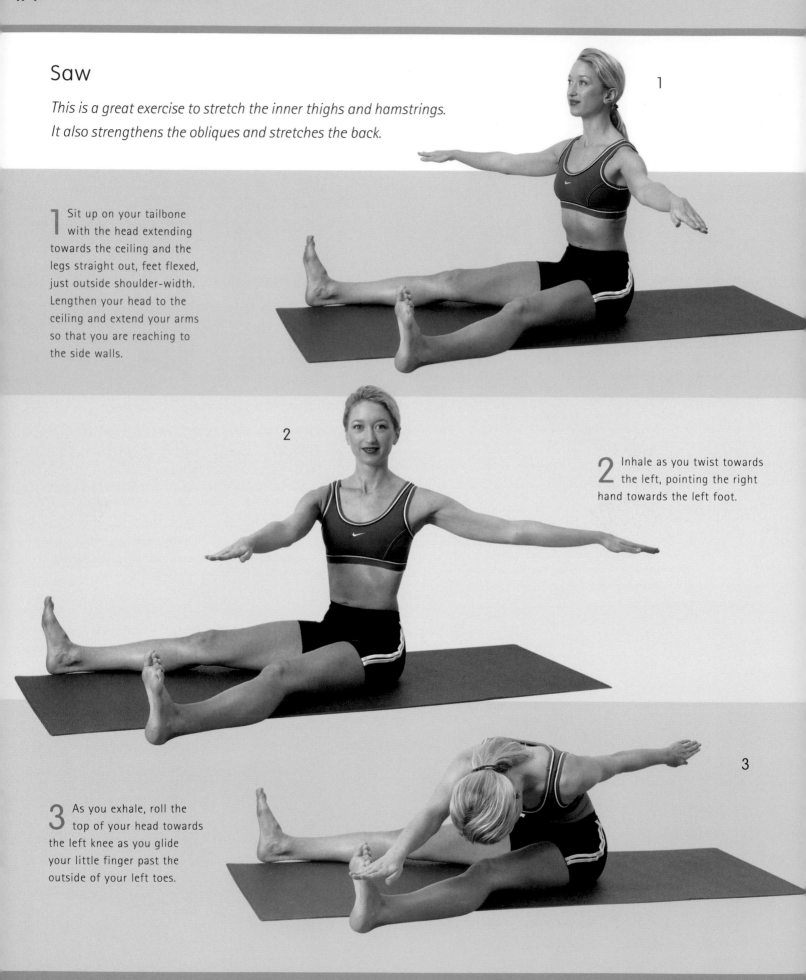

1 Sit up on your tailbone with the head extending towards the ceiling and the legs straight out, feet flexed, just outside shoulder-width. Lengthen your head to the ceiling and extend your arms so that you are reaching to the side walls.

2 Inhale as you twist towards the left, pointing the right hand towards the left foot.

3 As you exhale, roll the top of your head towards the left knee as you glide your little finger past the outside of your left toes.

4 As you inhale, roll up starting from the base of the spine, one vertebra at a time.

*This is an **original** **PILATES** *exercise**

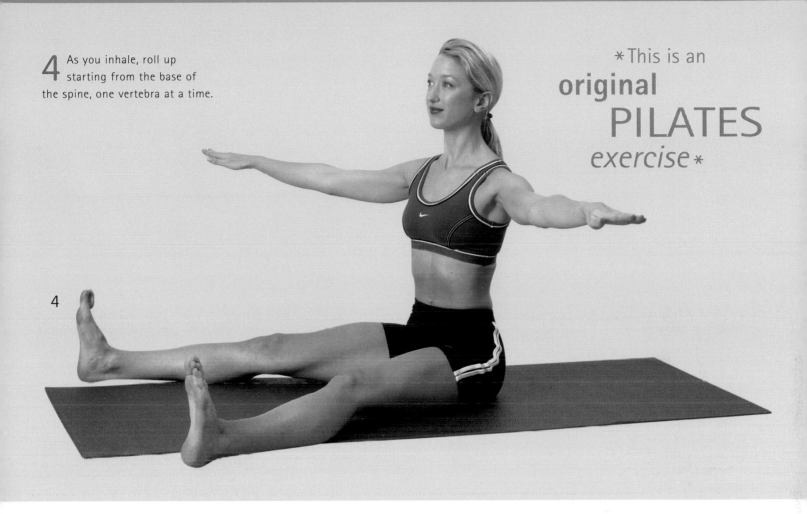

4

5 Exhale, rolling down to the right knee with your left hand gliding past your right toes.

6 Repeat three to four sets, counting the right and left side as one.

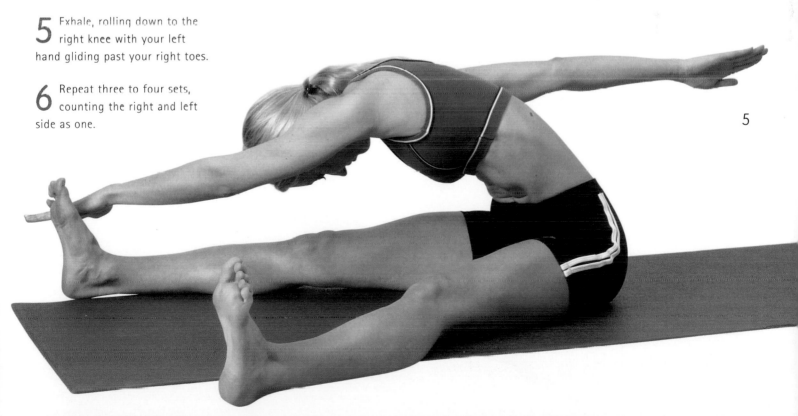

5

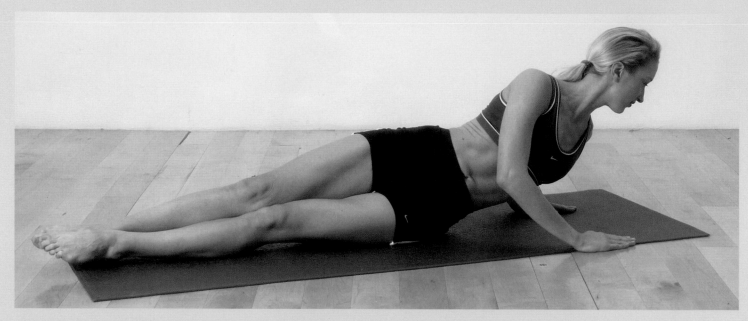

Transition: turn and place your hands on the mat to lie on your stomach for the Swan Dive.

Key Points:

- Make sure your hips stay anchored to the ground. Do not let the opposite hip come up as you roll forwards.

- Twist from the waistline.

- Think of the opposition as the tailbone presses down into the floor and your head lengthens in the opposite direction.

- Keep your shoulder blades pressing down the back and your neck long.

- Extend through the heels.

- Keep the knees and toes facing the ceiling.

Progression from:

Intermediate Saw, page 118.

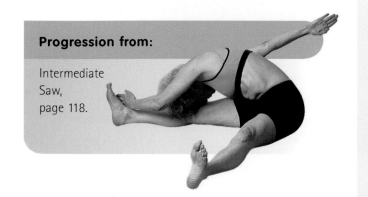

Modification:

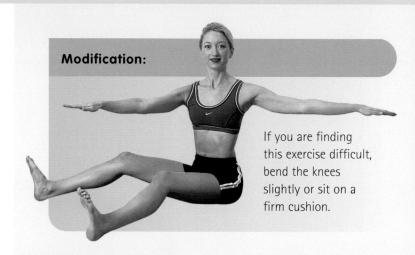

If you are finding this exercise difficult, bend the knees slightly or sit on a firm cushion.

Challenge:

You can grab the foot and lift it up, lean backwards slightly, and then place the foot down. Continue with the rest of the Saw as normal.

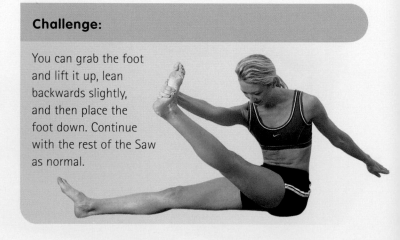

Swan Dive

The Swan Dive focuses on co-ordination of movement and strengthening and stretching the spine.

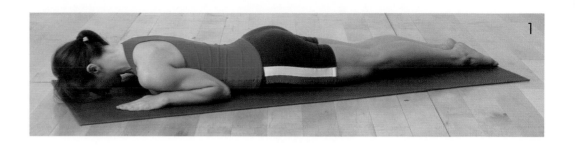

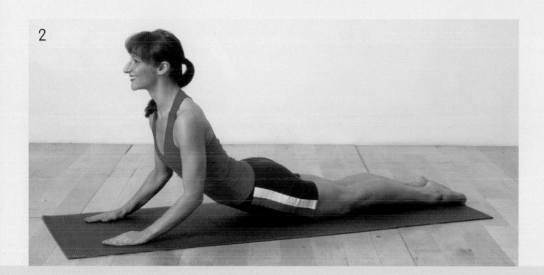

1 Lie on your stomach with your hands just outside your shoulders and your legs glued tight together.

2 Pull your navel into your spine and lengthen your head forwards as you straighten your arms, pressing your upper torso towards the ceiling.

3 Swing your arms forwards and rock from your abdominals as if you were a see-saw.

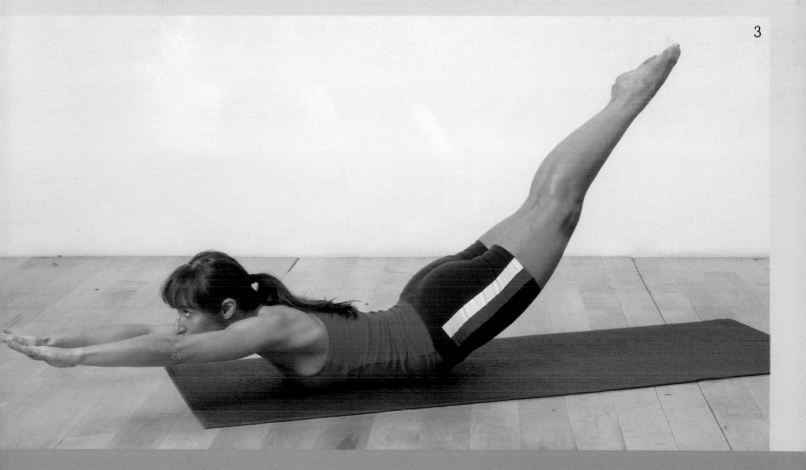

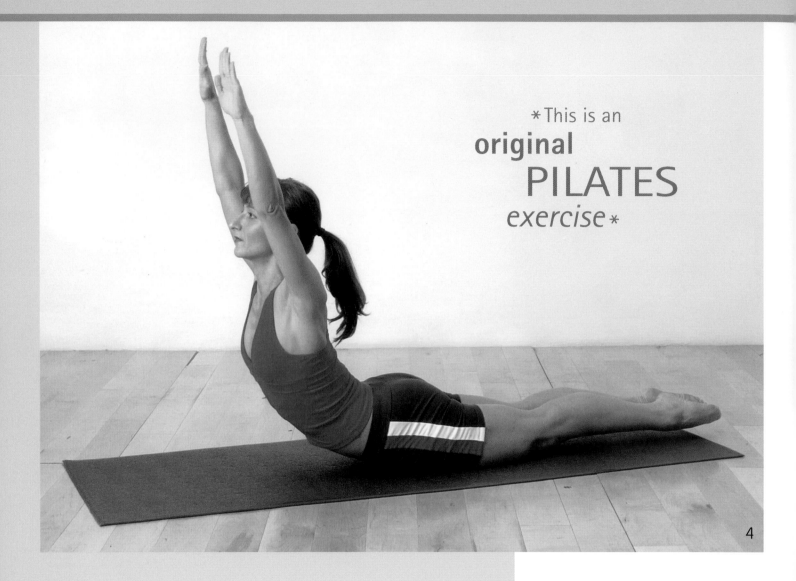

*This is an
original
PILATES
*exercise**

4

4 Inhale as the chest
comes up, exhale as the
legs come up. Repeat three
times.

5 Rest sitting on your
heels and stretching out
your spine (Child's Pose,
page 58).

5

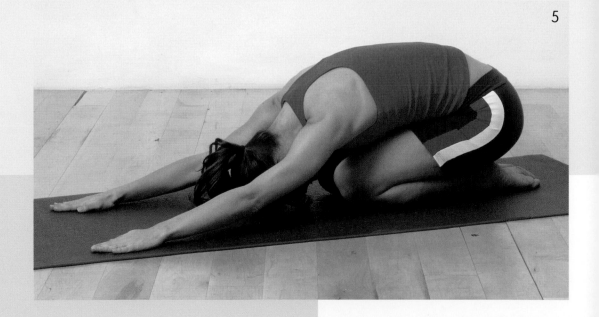

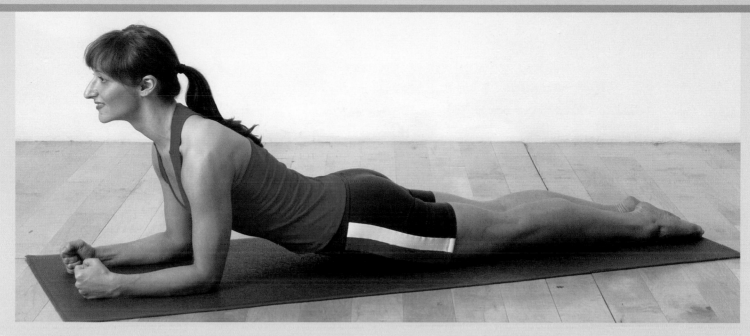

Transition: lie on your stomach with your legs straight and squeezed tight together. Prop yourself up on your elbows, with your fists in a straight line with your elbows, and your elbows in line with your shoulders, for the Single Leg Kicks.

Key Points:

- If you have problems with your back, please leave this exercise out.

- Keep pulling the navel into the spine and breathe through the sides and back of the ribs.

- Do not throw the arms or the feet.

- Try to roll evenly through the body and in a straight line.

- Keep your legs glued together throughout the movement.

Modification:

Baby Swan Dive

1 Lie on your stomach. Place the hands under your head with your elbows out to the sides. Inhale to prepare.

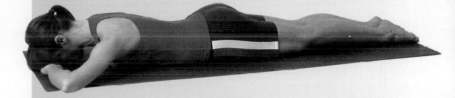

2 As you exhale pull the stomach off the mat. Inhale to relax. On the second exhale, lift the legs and torso off the mat. Repeat five times, continuing to pull the navel into the spine.

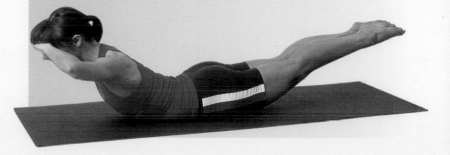

Progression from:

Shoulder Blades, page 55.

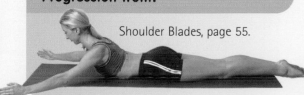

Single Leg Kicks

This exercise is for rhythm, strengthening the upper body, hamstrings and buttocks, while stretching the quadriceps.

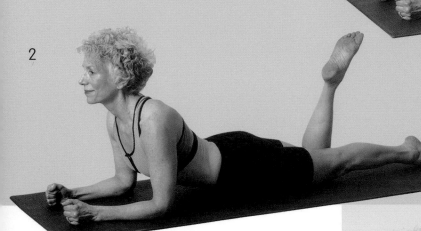

1

1 Lie on your stomach with your legs straight and squeezed tightly together. Prop yourself up on your elbows, with your fists in a straight line with your elbows, and your elbows in line with your shoulders. Looking directly in front of you, pull your navel and ribcage up so that the stomach barely touches the mat. Squeeze your buttocks.

2

2 Bend one leg and kick your buttocks twice.

3 Switch legs passing them in the air, and kick twice with the opposite leg.

4 Counting the right and left as one, repeat six to ten times.

5 Breathe naturally for the whole exercise.

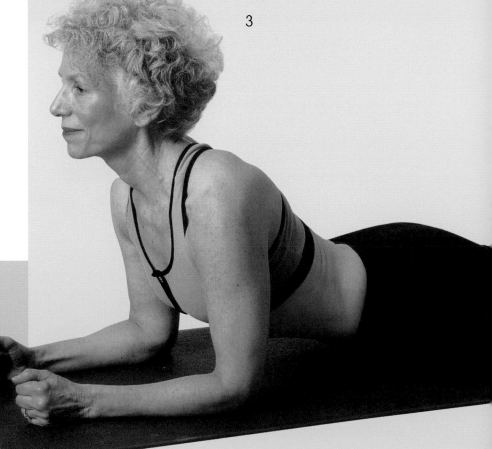

3

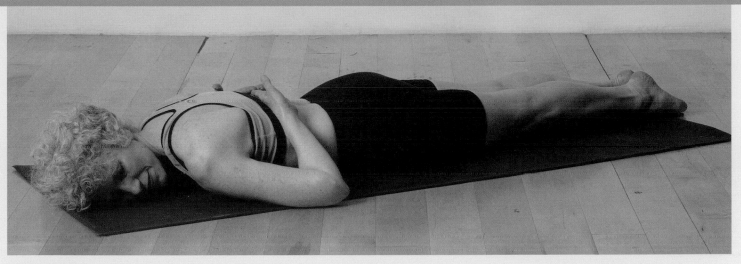

Transition: lie on your stomach and clasp one hand in the other. Place the hands high on the back and press the elbows down on the floor. You are now ready for Double Leg Kicks.

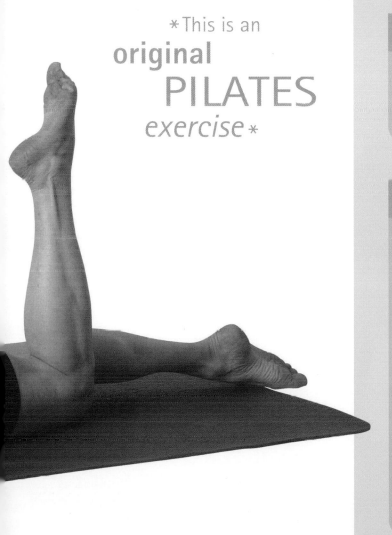

*This is an
original
PILATES
*exercise**

Key Points:

- Make sure you keep the lower back long and the shoulders down.

- Lift up and out of your hips.

- Keep the buttocks and knees squeezed tightly throughout.

Challenge:

Once you have mastered this exercise, on the two kicks into the buttocks, try: a) pointing for one kick, and b) flexing for the other.

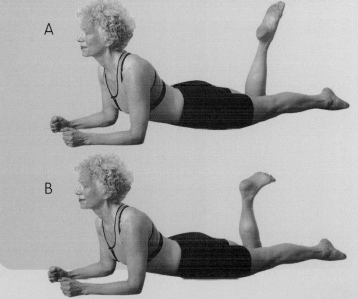

A

B

Double Leg Kicks

This exercise is great for strengthening the buttocks and hamstrings, and stretching the chest, upper back and arms.

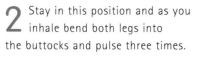

1 Lie on your stomach on the floor with your legs out straight and clasp one hand in the other high behind your back. Hold the fingers of one hand with the other and try to pull the elbows down to the floor. Look to the left so the right cheek is on the mat.

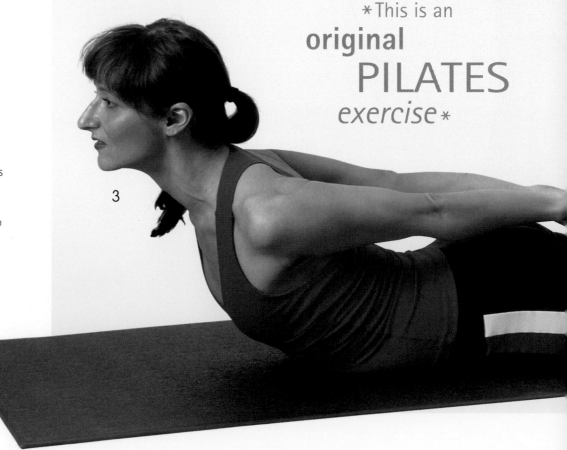

2 Stay in this position and as you inhale bend both legs into the buttocks and pulse three times.

3 As you exhale, straighten your legs, and extend your arms towards the pelvis and lift the chest and head off the floor.

4 As you relax back down, look to the right so that the left cheek is on the mat.

5 Repeat the whole exercise two to three more times.

*This is an
original
PILATES
*exercise**

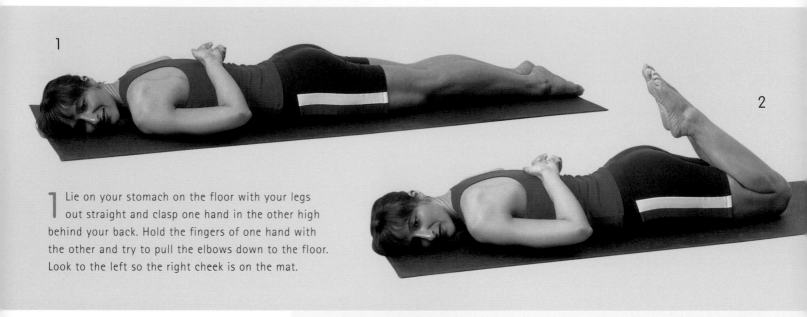

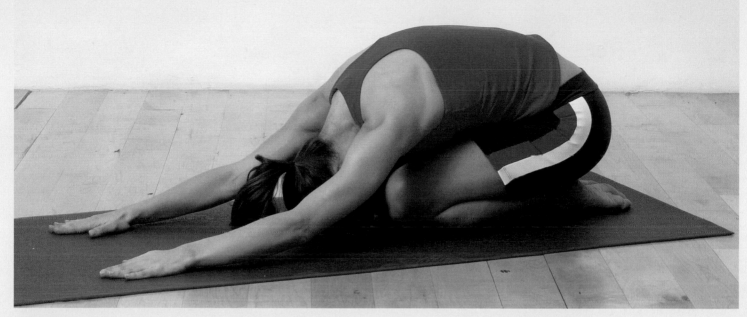

Transition: bring your buttocks back to sit on your heels. Relax the upper torso forwards for the Rest Position.

Key Points:

- If you have problems with your back, please leave this exercise out.

- Keep the elbows reaching towards the floor as you kick your feet towards your buttocks.

- Keep the navel into the spine to support your lower back.

- Keep your neck long as you reach your hands towards your feet and lift the chest up.

- Keep your buttocks squeezed tightly throughout.

Challenge:

Try reversing the breath once you have mastered this exercise.

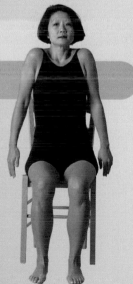

Progression from:

Shoulder Shrugs, page 38

Buttocks Squeeze, page 54.

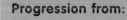

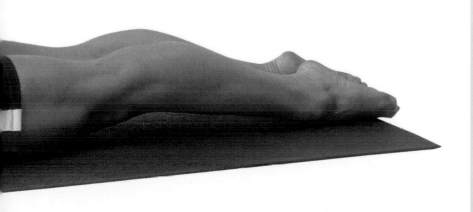

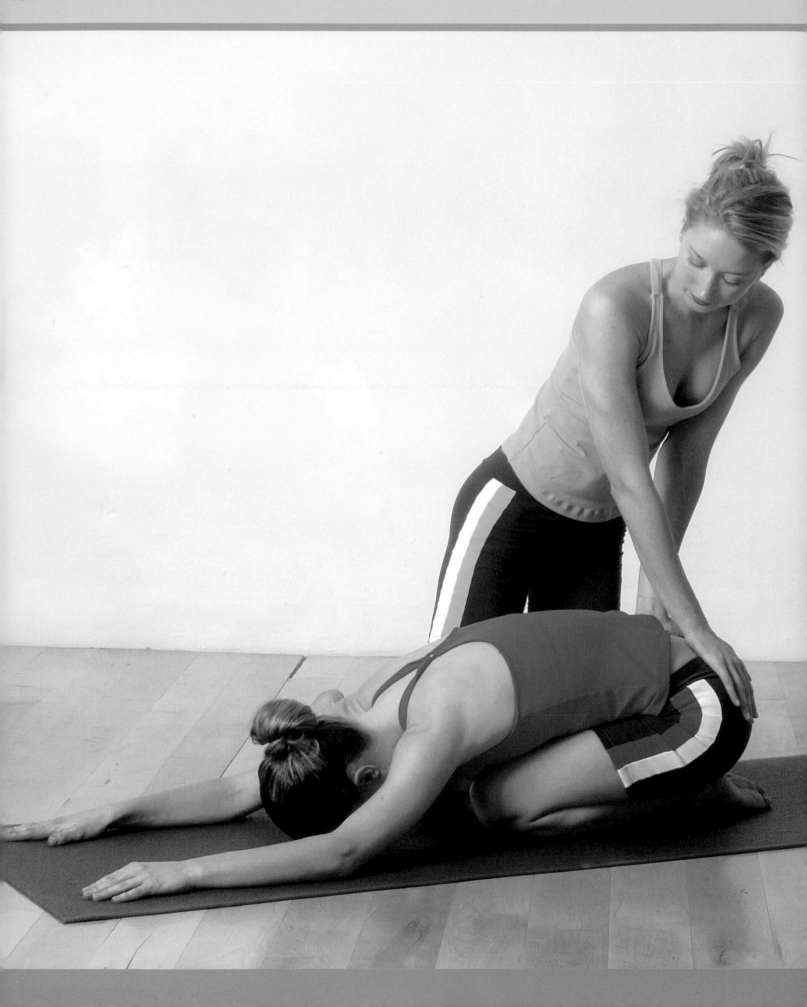

Rest Position

The Rest Position is a lovely stretch on the back and arms.

1 Sit on your heels and extend your upper torso forwards so that the arms are long and reaching away from you on the mat. Keep your head relaxed on the mat. Take three deep breaths, stretching out the spine.

2 Slowly roll up to a sitting position.

Key Points:

- If you have problems with your knees, please leave this exercise out.

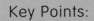

Transition: cross the ankles as you sit back on the pelvis. Extend your legs hip-width apart as you roll backwards and lace your hands behind your head for the Neck Pull.

1
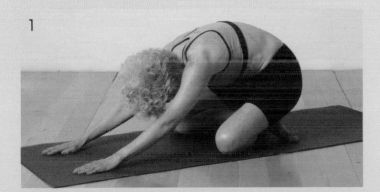

3
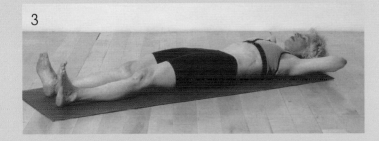

2
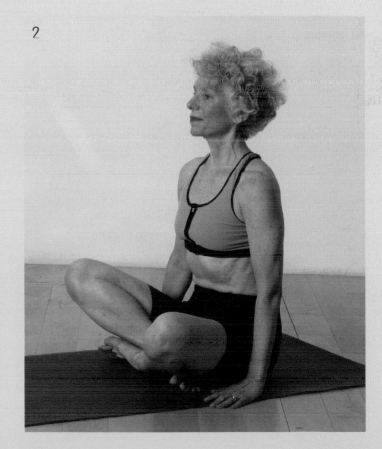

Neck Pull

The Neck Pull strengthens your abdominals and stretches your lower back and hamstrings. Focus on co-ordination, control and flow of movement.

1 Lie on your back with your legs extended straight along the mat, hip-width apart. Lace your fingers behind your head with your elbows slightly lifted off the mat.

2 As you inhale, round up to a sitting position.

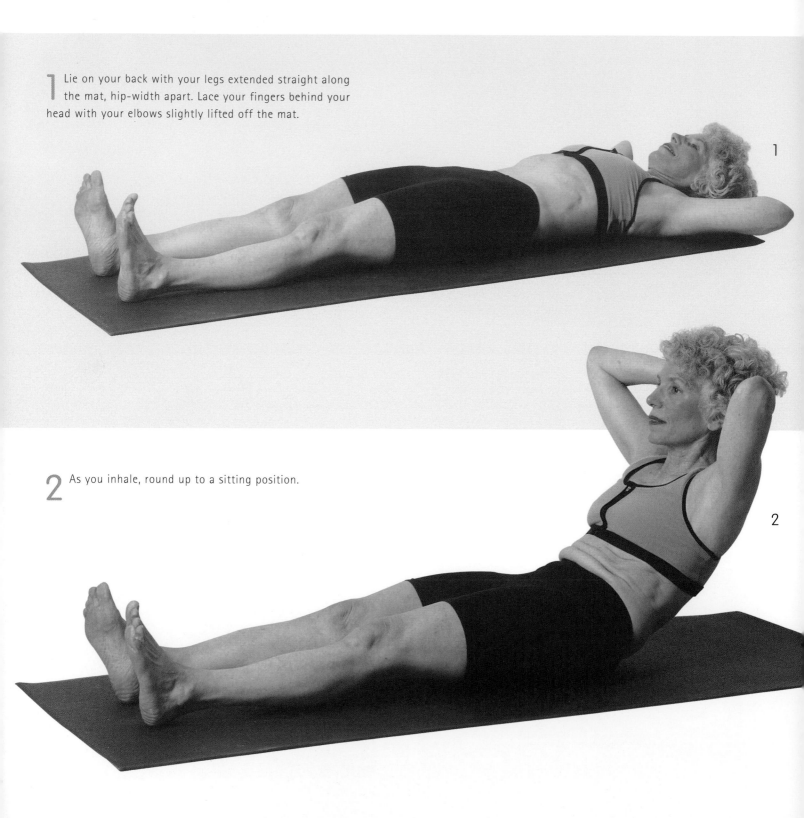

3 As you exhale, round forwards, trying to bring your head between your knees. Your elbows should be on the outside of the knees, and your head on the inside of the knees.

4 Inhale to a tall, flat back.

5 Exhale and curl the tailbone forwards lengthening the back down, vertebra by vertebra.

6 Repeat five times.

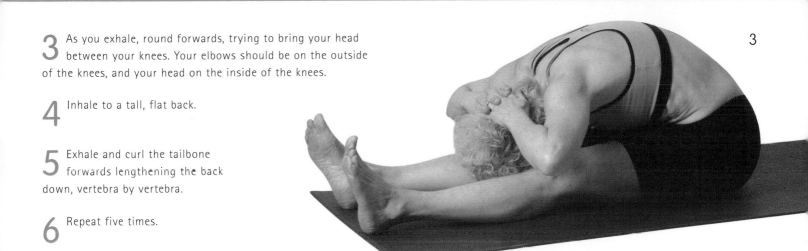
3

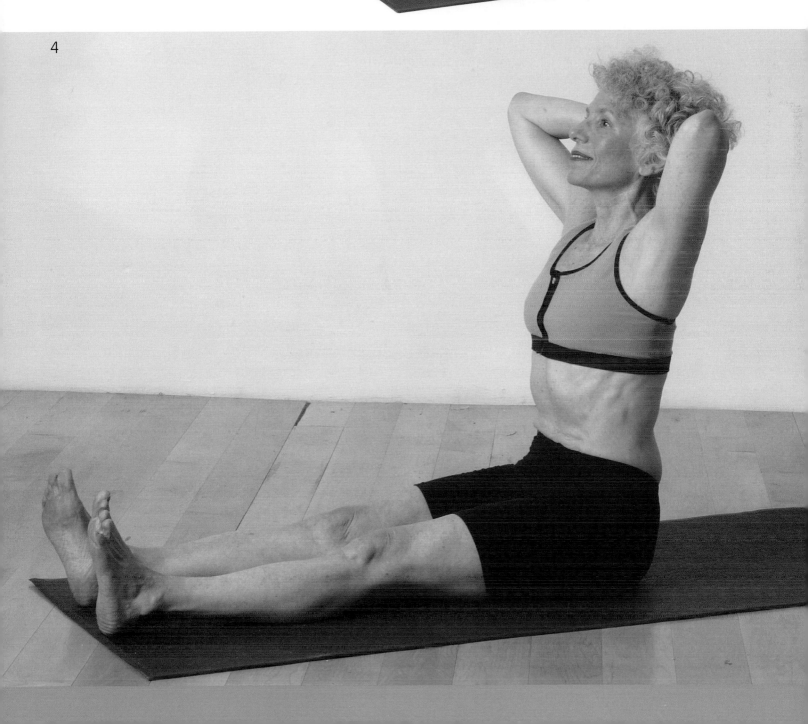
4

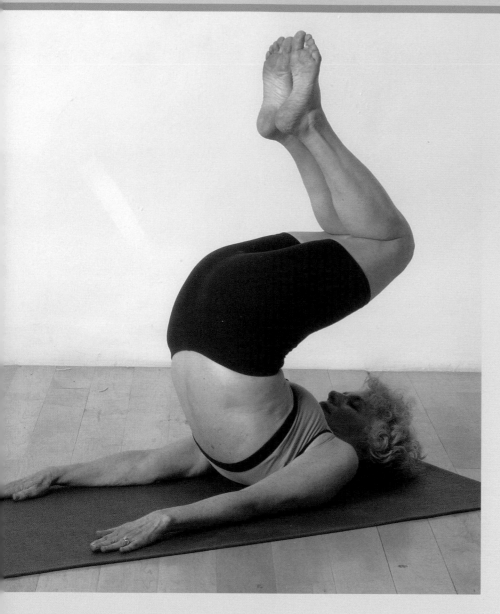

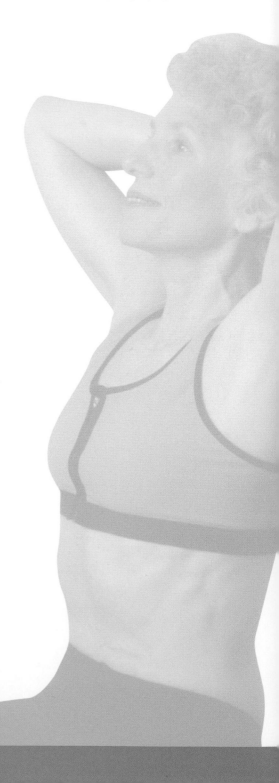

*This is an
original
PILATES
*exercise**

Transition: lie on your back, bend your knees and roll up on to your shoulders to start Scissors.

Key Points:

- Make sure you are not leading with one shoulder.

- Extend through the heels.

- Keep the shoulder blades pulling down the back.

- Keep the navel pulling into the spine and breathe through the sides and back of the ribs.

- Do not let the feet fly off the mat.

Modification:

Basic Roll-up. page 92.

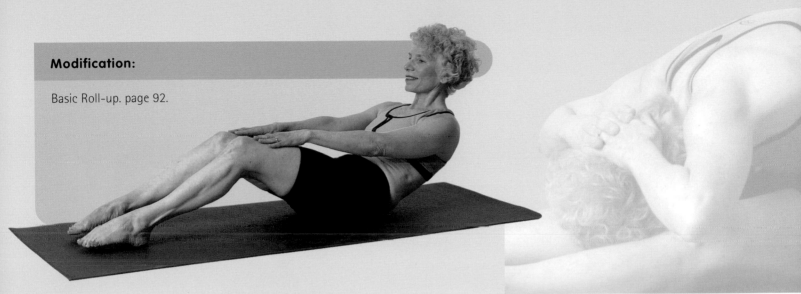

Challenge 1:

After step 4, lengthen with a flat back as far as you can control. Start rolling down from tailbone when necessary.

Challenge 2:

After you complete step 2, exhale and twist, touching the elbow to opposite knee, then the other, then sit up tall and complete the exercise as normal.

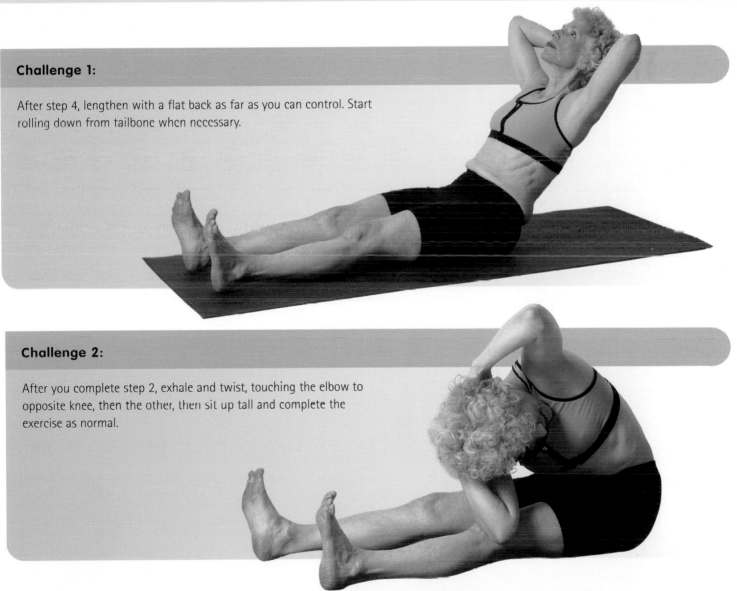

Scissors

The Scissors concentrates on opening the hips, while strengthening and stretching the quadriceps and hamstrings. It is important to focus on balance, co-ordination and rhythm.

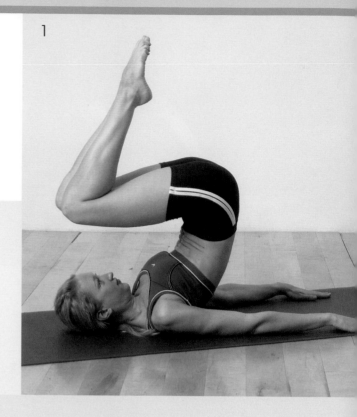

1 Lie on your back, bend your knees into your chest and push up so your pelvis is in the air and you are resting on your shoulder blades.

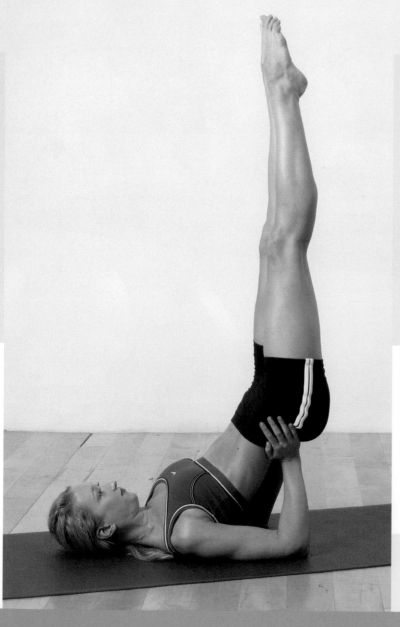

2 Place one hand underneath each hip, with the fingers facing outwards and the elbows directly under the hands. Relax the pelvis into the hands and extend the legs towards the ceiling.

3 Keeping the left foot in line with the eyes, pulse the right leg towards the floor twice.

4 Let the legs pass in the air, and pulse the left leg towards the floor twice.

5 Repeat five times.

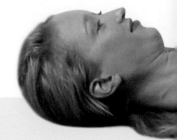

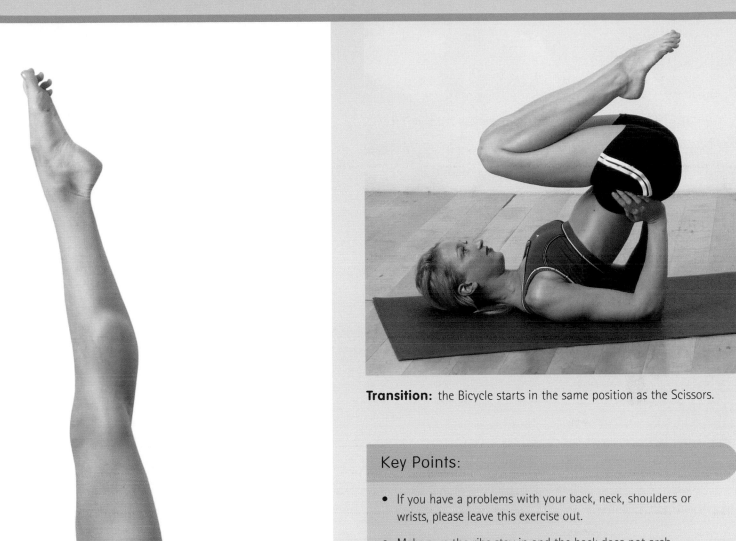

Transition: the Bicycle starts in the same position as the Scissors.

Key Points:

- If you have a problems with your back, neck, shoulders or wrists, please leave this exercise out.

- Make sure the ribs stay in and the back does not arch.

- Extend through the toes.

- Keep the legs straight throughout.

*This is an
original PILATES
*exercise**

Bicycle

The Bicycle is very similar to the Scissors and also focuses on opening the hips while strengthening and stretching the hamstrings. Focus on balance, co-ordination and rhythm.

1 Start in the same position as the Scissors. Lie on your back, bend your knees into your chest and push up so your pelvis is in the air and you are resting on your shoulder blades. Place one hand underneath each hip, with the fingers facing outwards and the elbows directly under the hands. Relax the pelvis into the hands and extend the legs towards the ceiling.

2 Think of riding an imaginary bicycle. Extend your left leg up to the ceiling then down towards the floor.

*This is an **original** PILATES *exercise* *

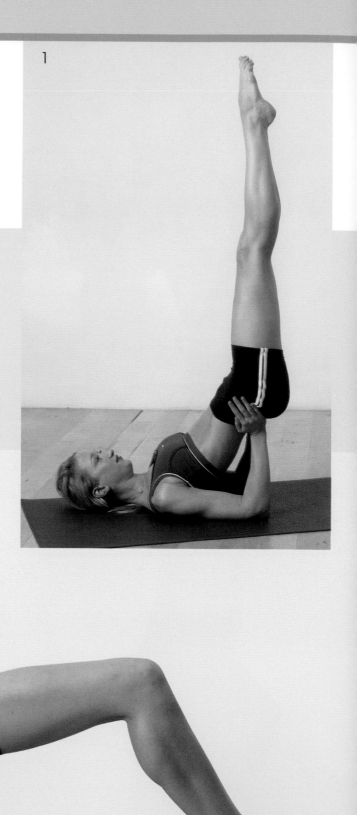

1

2

3

3 As you bend it back in, start extending the right leg up towards the ceiling and out towards the floor.

4 Repeat three times and then reverse, riding your imaginary bicycle backwards three times.

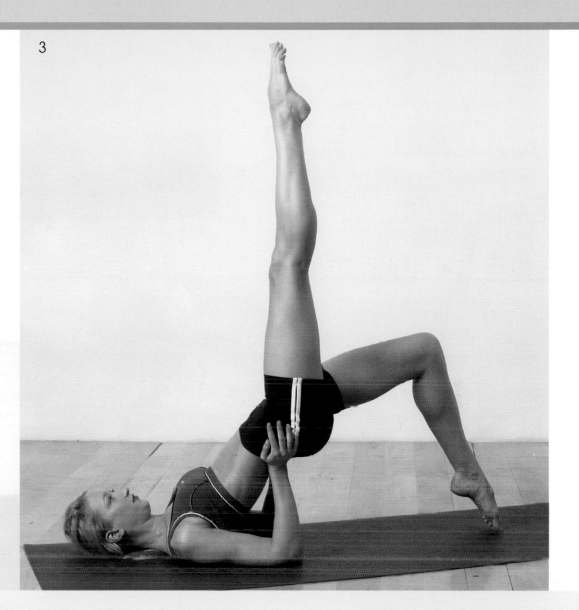

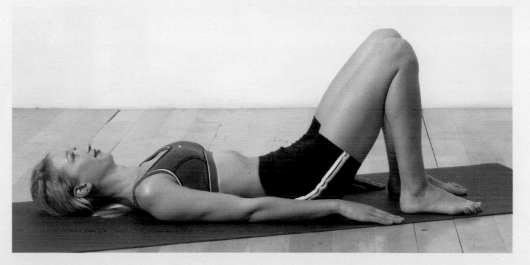

Key Points:

- If you have problems with your back, neck, shoulders or wrists, please leave this exercise out.

- Make sure the ribs stay in and the back does not arch.

- Extend through the toes.

Transition: relax the arms to the sides and roll down sequentially through the spine. Bend your knees and place the feet flat on the floor hip-width apart to prepare for the Shoulder Bridge.

Shoulder Bridge

The Shoulder Bridge focuses on mobility of the spine, while strengthening and stretching the hamstrings and buttocks. Think of initiating the movement from your powerhouse.

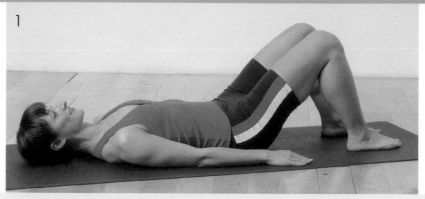

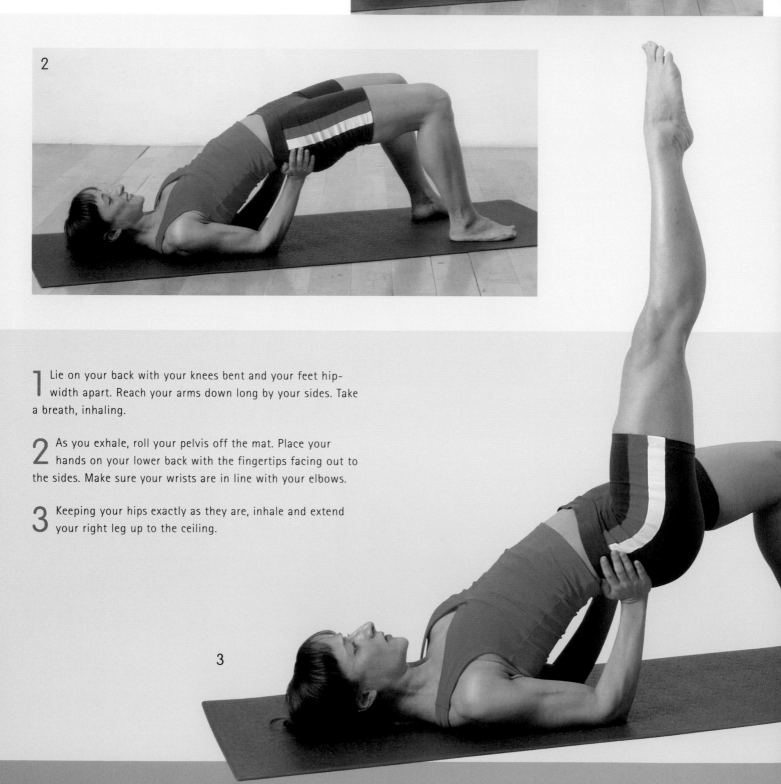

1 Lie on your back with your knees bent and your feet hip-width apart. Reach your arms down long by your sides. Take a breath, inhaling.

2 As you exhale, roll your pelvis off the mat. Place your hands on your lower back with the fingertips facing out to the sides. Make sure your wrists are in line with your elbows.

3 Keeping your hips exactly as they are, inhale and extend your right leg up to the ceiling.

4 As you exhale, flex the toes and bring the straight leg down to the mat.

5 The leg should stay in line with your hip socket.

6 As you inhale, point the foot and kick it back up towards the ceiling. Repeat five times on the right side.

7 Keeping the hips high, change legs and repeat on the other side.

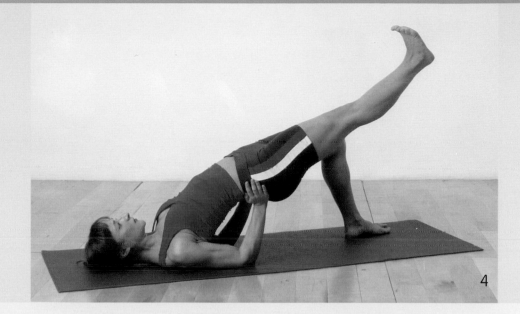

4

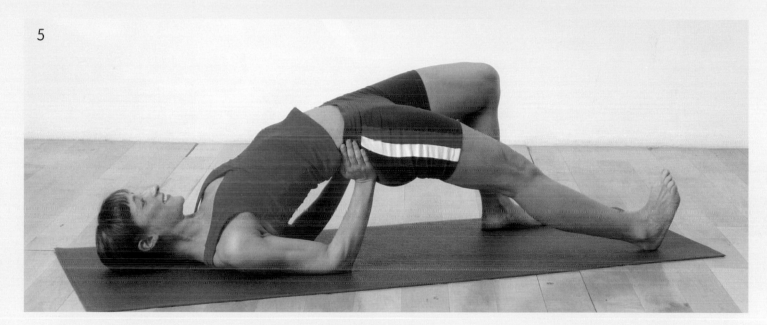

5

Progression from:

Pelvic Curl with Leg Lifts, page 64.

Challenge:

Leg Pull-up, page 224.

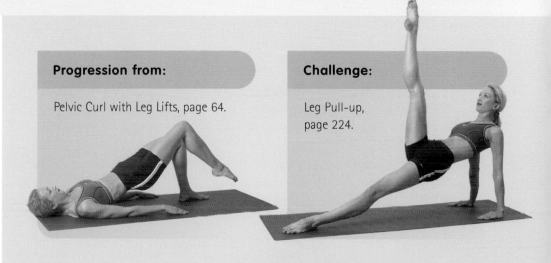

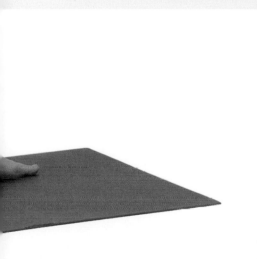

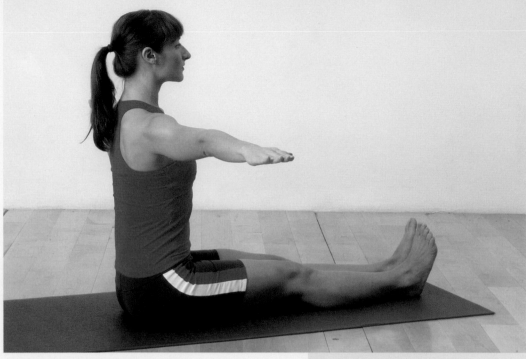

*This is an
original
PILATES
*exercise**

Transition: relax the arms down by your sides and roll down your spine, vertebra by vertebra. Extend your legs straight as you round up to a sitting position. Lengthen your head towards the ceiling as you extend your arms out to the sides. Squeeze your legs together and flex the feet for the Spine Twist.

Key Points:

- Make sure the hips, knees and feet stay in alignment the whole time.

- Do not let the hips drop and lift with the movement of the leg.

- Keep the navel pulling into the spine and breathe through the back and sides of the ribs.

- Keep the shoulders down and the neck long.

- Keep the ribs in throughout the exercise.

Modification:

If you are putting strain on your arms and back, relax the arms down by your side and lower your hips a little. Continue with the exercise as normal.

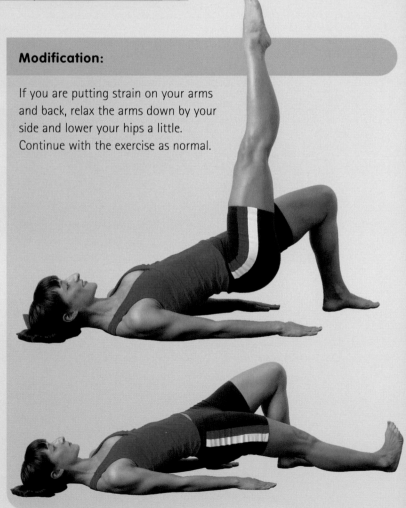

1

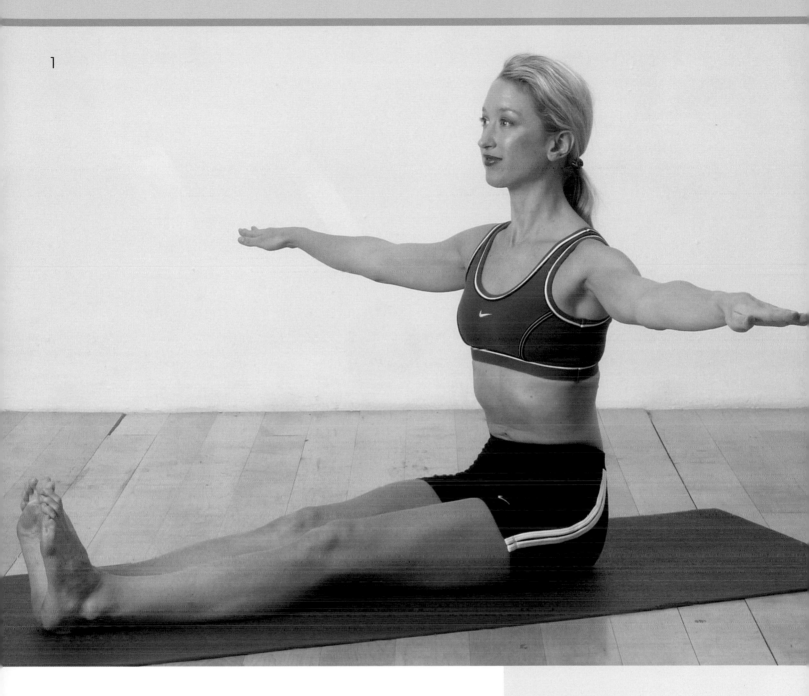

Spine Twist

The Spine Twist is the next progression of the Beginner's Twist on page 44. It focuses on lengthening and stretching the spine, while wringing out the lungs. Think of lifting the ribcage away from the hips, while keeping the back long and pulling the shoulder blades down.

1 Sit up with the legs straight and glued tight together. Extend the arms, reaching towards the side walls, and flex the feet. The head is lengthening towards the ceiling and the heels are pressing away. Inhale to stay.

2   As you exhale, keep your back straight and tall as if
    lifting up out of the hips and twist from the ribcage,
pulsing to the left twice.

3   Inhale bringing the torso to face the feet again,
    keeping the arms on the back.

2

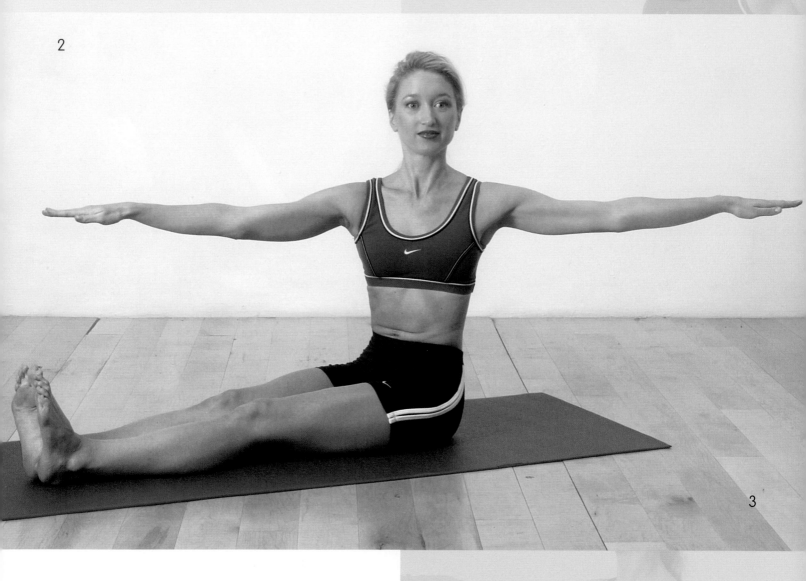

3

4   As you exhale for the second time, twist from the
    ribcage pulsing to the right twice.

5   Repeat four times to each side.

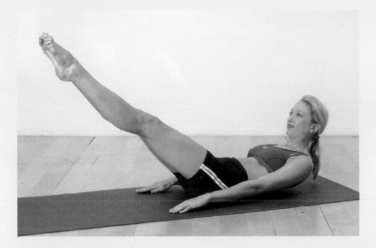 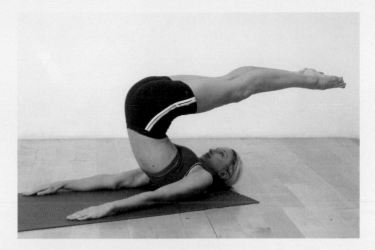

Transition: relax the arms down by your side and roll on to your back, one vertebra at a time. Pull your abdominals in, lift your legs straight off the mat and roll on to the shoulders with the legs parallel to the ground behind you to prepare for the Jackknife.

Key Points:

- Make sure the back is flat and the legs are straight and glued tight together.

- Think of the chest being open and the shoulders down the whole time.

- Keep your feet in one line and extend through the heels.

- Twist from the waistline.

- Keep the navel pulling into the spine and breathe through the sides and back of the ribs.

- Think of lengthening through your tailbone and the top of your head while extending the hands out to the side walls.

- Keep the shoulder blades pulling down the back.

*This is an
original PILATES
exercise*

Modification:

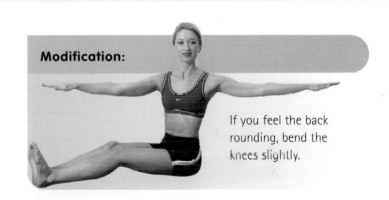

If you feel the back rounding, bend the knees slightly.

Progression from:

Beginner's Twist, page 44; and Intermediate Bent Leg Spine Twist, page 120.

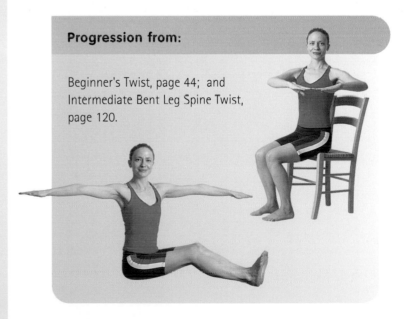

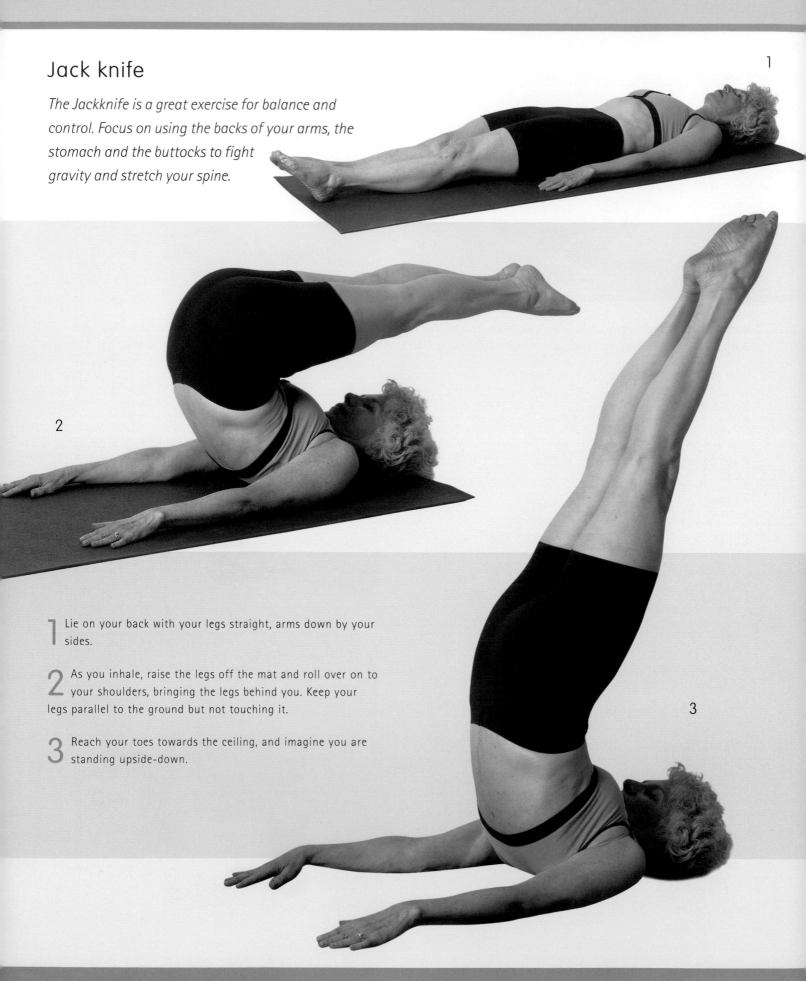

Jack knife

The Jackknife is a great exercise for balance and control. Focus on using the backs of your arms, the stomach and the buttocks to fight gravity and stretch your spine.

1. Lie on your back with your legs straight, arms down by your sides.

2. As you inhale, raise the legs off the mat and roll over on to your shoulders, bringing the legs behind you. Keep your legs parallel to the ground but not touching it.

3. Reach your toes towards the ceiling, and imagine you are standing upside-down.

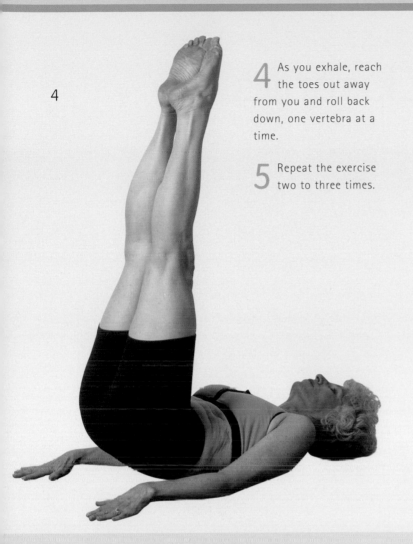

4

4 As you exhale, reach the toes out away from you and roll back down, one vertebra at a time.

5 Repeat the exercise two to three times.

Key Points:

- If you have problems with your neck or back, please leave this exercise out.

- Keep the navel pulling into the spine and breathe through the sides and back of your ribs.

- Keep the buttocks and inner thighs squeezed throughout.

- Try to make this exercise smooth and continuous.

- Extend through the toes.

- Roll up on to the shoulders and not the neck.

- Press the palms into the floor to aid stabilization.

*This is an
original PILATES
exercise *

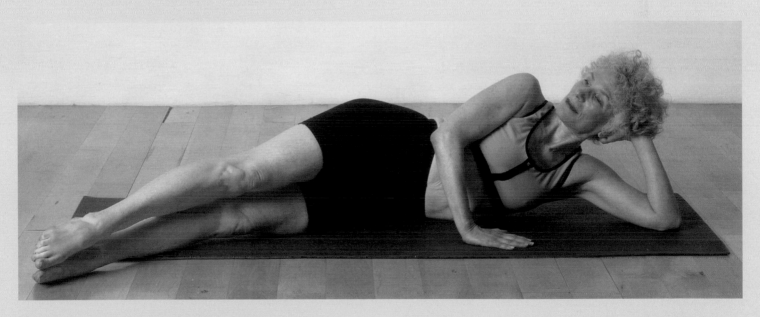

Transition: lie on your left side with your head in your hand, right hand pressing into the floor in front of your chest. Make sure the shoulders and hips are in line and your legs are at a slight diagonal in front to prepare for the Side Kick series.

Side Kick series

The next four exercises are performed together. Lying on your right side, do the Side Kicks, Ronde de Jambe, Bicycle on Side and Taps on the left side before turning over on to your right side to repeat the exercises.

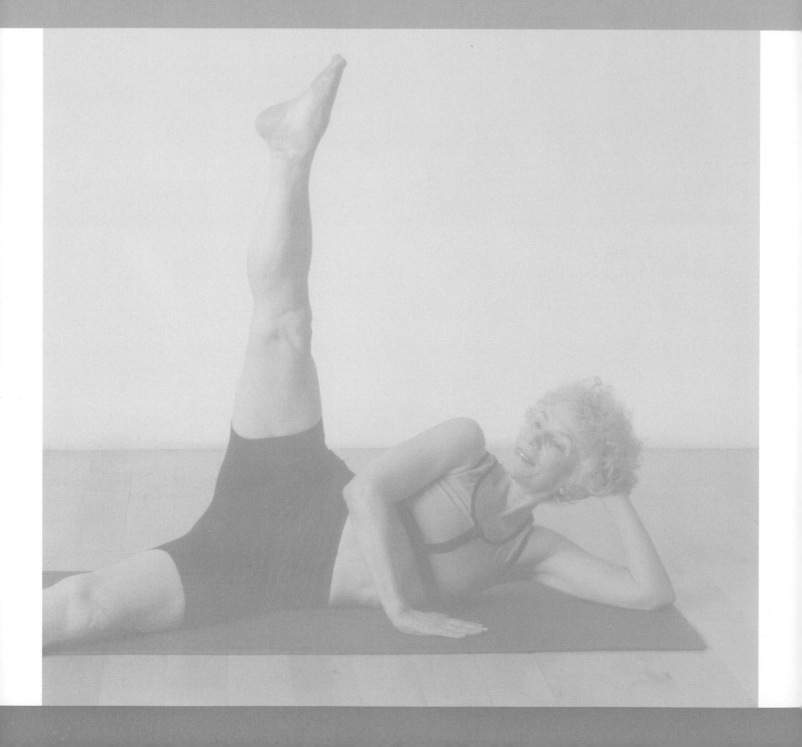

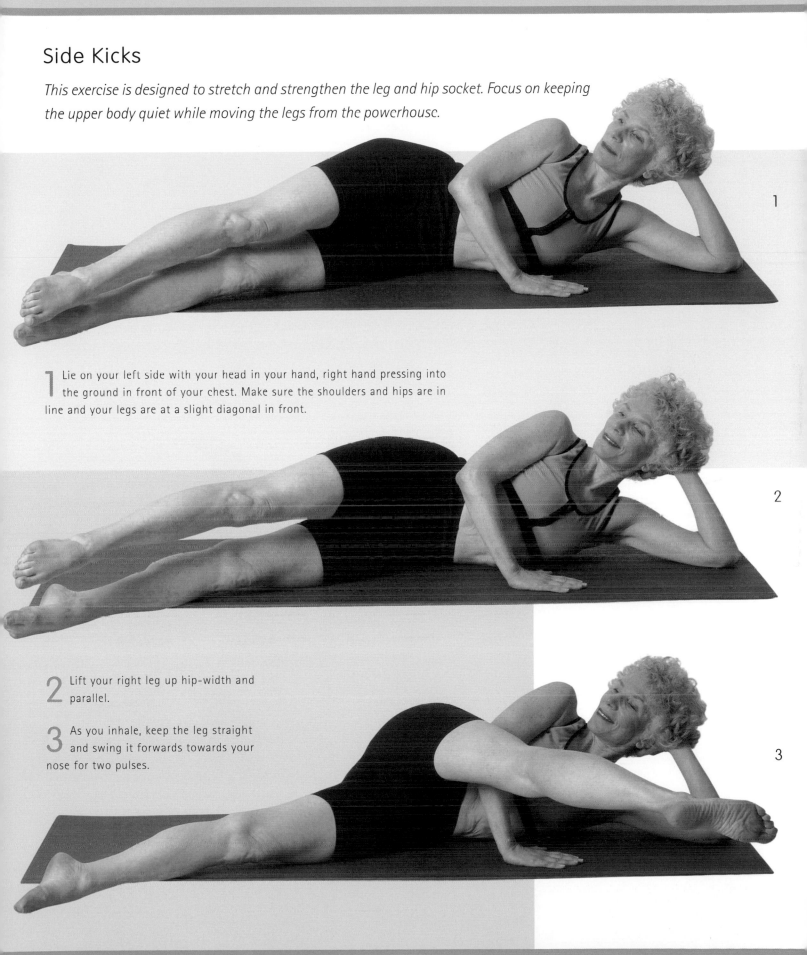

Side Kicks

This exercise is designed to stretch and strengthen the leg and hip socket. Focus on keeping the upper body quiet while moving the legs from the powerhouse.

1 Lie on your left side with your head in your hand, right hand pressing into the ground in front of your chest. Make sure the shoulders and hips are in line and your legs are at a slight diagonal in front.

2 Lift your right leg up hip-width and parallel.

3 As you inhale, keep the leg straight and swing it forwards towards your nose for two pulses.

4

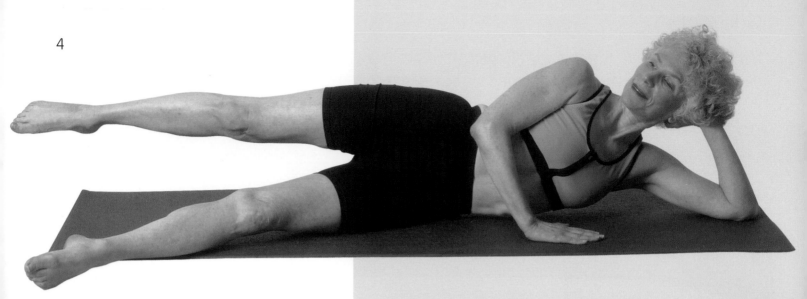

4 As you exhale, swing the leg back with two pulses.

5 Repeat a total of ten times.

Transition: remain in the same place for the Ronde de Jambe.

Key Points:

- Make sure the upper torso does not move.

- Keep the leg hip-width the whole time.

- Keep the top hip directly over the bottom hip the whole time. Do not let the hip move forwards or backwards.

- Keep the movement as small as you need to for stability.

Challenge:

After you have mastered this exercise, try placing both hands behind your head with the elbows long and wide.

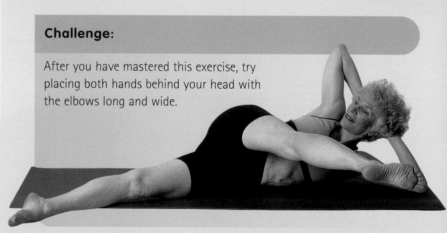

Variation:

Flex the foot to the front and point the foot to the back.

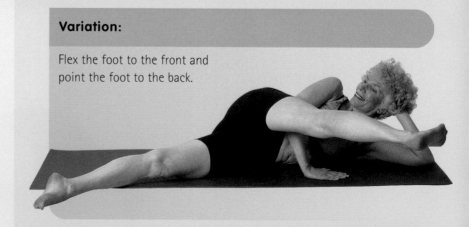

*This is an
original PILATES
exercise *

Ronde de Jambe

This exercise is designed to stretch and strengthen the leg while opening the hip socket. Focus on keeping the hips still while moving the leg.

1

1 Lie on your left side with your head relaxed in your left hand. The right hand should be placed lightly on the ground in front of you. Make sure the shoulders and hips are in line and your feet are slightly on the diagonal in front.

2 Lift your right leg up hip-width and turn it out so that the knee is facing the ceiling.

3

3 Inhale as the right leg circles forwards towards your nose.

4 Lift the leg towards the ceiling and rotate it back behind you as you exhale. Do not let the hips move forwards or backwards.

5 Repeat three times in this direction, and then immediately reverse directions.

4

Key Points:

- Make sure the upper torso does not move.

- Keep the top hip directly over the bottom hip the whole time. Do not let the hip move forwards or backwards.

- Keep the movement as small as you need to for stability.

5

This is an
original
PILATES
exercise *

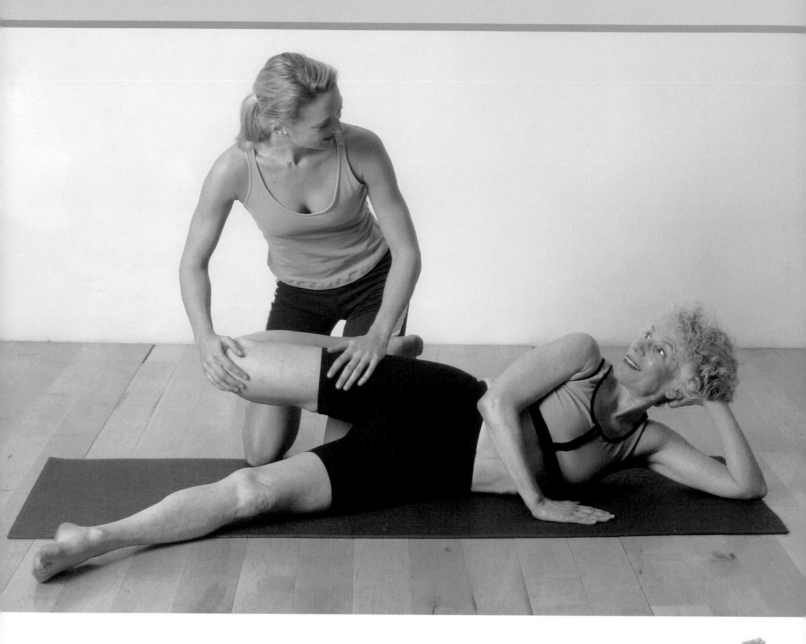

Bicycle on Side

This is a great exercise to strengthen the hip socket, while stretching the hamstrings and quadriceps.

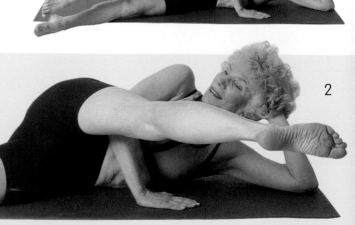

1

1 Lie on your left side with your head relaxed in your hand. Make sure your shoulders and hips are in one line and your feet are slightly in front on a low diagonal.

2 Lift your right leg to hip-height and parallel to the floor.

2

3 Swing the leg forwards towards your nose. Keep the knee in this position while bringing the foot towards your buttocks.

4 Keeping the foot close to the buttocks, swing the knee back behind you without letting it drop.

3

4

5 Again, keeping the knee where it is in space, extend the foot out.

6 Repeat three times.

7 To reverse: swing the leg back behind you without letting your upper torso move.

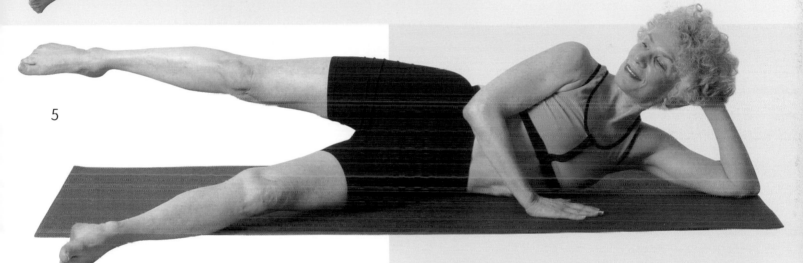

5

8 Keep the knee in this position while bringing the foot towards your buttocks.

9 Keeping the foot close to the buttocks, swing the knee towards the shoulder without letting it drop.

10 Again, keeping the knee where it is in space, extend the foot out.

11 Repeat three times.

Transition: you are already in position for Taps.

Key Points:

• If you have problems with your knees, please leave this exercise out.

• Make sure the upper torso does not move.

• Keep the top hip directly over the bottom hip the whole time. Do not let the hip move forwards or backwards.

• Keep the movement as small as you need to for stability

*This is an
original PILATES
exercise*

Taps

This is a great exercise is for rhythm, control and flexibility of the hips. Concentrate on precise, accurate movements of the leg.

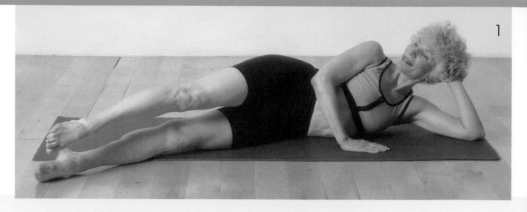

1

2

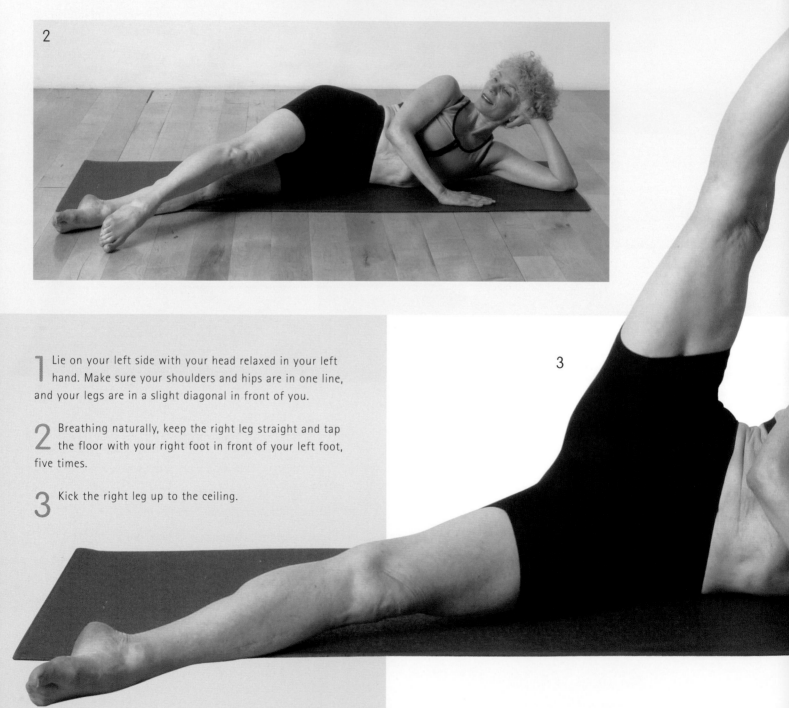

1 Lie on your left side with your head relaxed in your left hand. Make sure your shoulders and hips are in one line, and your legs are in a slight diagonal in front of you.

2 Breathing naturally, keep the right leg straight and tap the floor with your right foot in front of your left foot, five times.

3 Kick the right leg up to the ceiling.

3

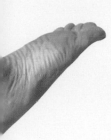
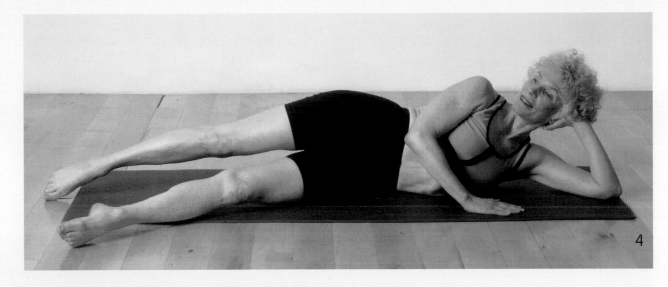

4

4 Then tap the floor to the back of the left leg five times..

5 Kick the leg back up towards the ceiling.

6 Repeat the sequence with four taps.

7 Repeat the sequence with three taps, then two taps, then one tap.

8 Repeat the whole side kick series to the other side.

Transition: roll on to your back with your legs extended and your arms reaching overhead with your ribcage down to prepare for Teasers.

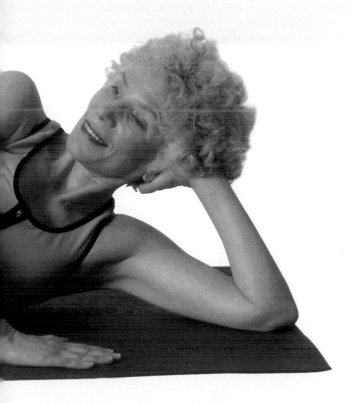

Key Points:

- Make sure the upper torso does not move.

- Keep the top hip directly over the bottom hip the whole time. Do not let the hip move forwards or backwards.

- Keep the movement as small as you need to for stability

*This is an
original PILATES
exercise

Teaser 1

The Teaser 1 is a fun exercise working on balance and co-ordination. It also focuses on strengthening the abdominals, inner thighs and hip flexors.

1 Lie on your back with your arms overhead and reaching straight out. Pull your navel into your spine and raise your legs straight to a 45-degree angle, toes apart and heels together.

2 As you inhale, raise the arms to the ceiling. Lift the chin into the chest and slowly curl forwards, rolling up vertebra by vertebra until the hands are reaching towards the feet (Teaser position). Make sure the legs do not move.

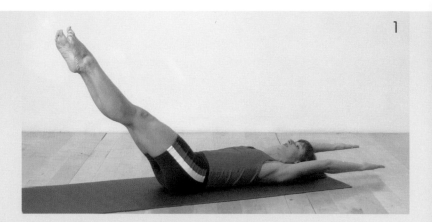

1

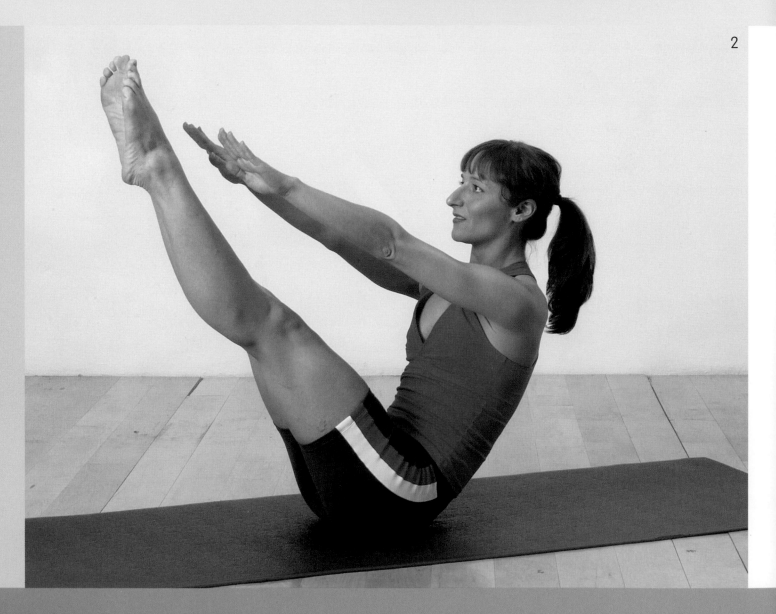

2

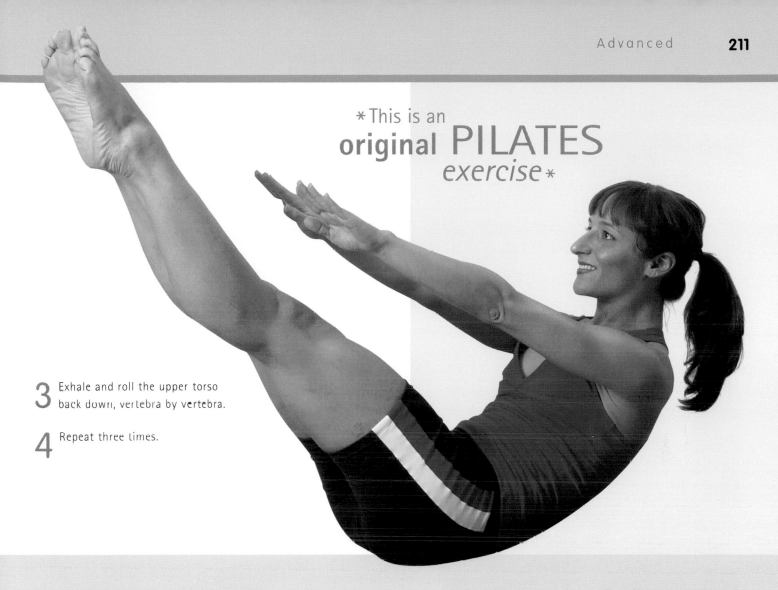

*This is an
original PILATES
exercise *

3 Exhale and roll the upper torso back down, vertebra by vertebra.

4 Repeat three times.

Transition: start another Teaser 1 and after you reach step 2, stay there and you are ready for Teaser 2.

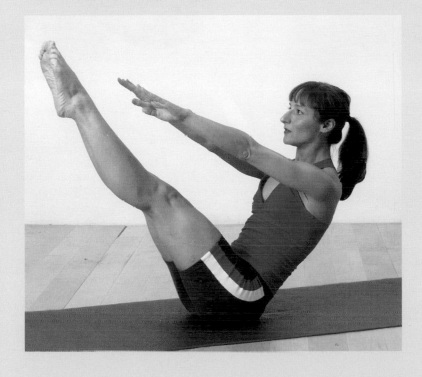

Key Points:

- If you have a problems with your back, please leave this exercise out.

- Make sure the back rolls up and down sequentially.

- Keep the navel pulling into the spine and breathe through the back and sides of the ribs.

- Keep the shoulder blades pulling down the back.

- Lengthen through the toes and reach out through the fingertips.

- Glue the inner thighs together and squeeze the buttocks.

- If your back starts to arch please stop this exercise.

- Keep the legs straight and in one place in space all the time. Do not let the legs lower and lift.

- Do not arch! Do not let the arms whip!

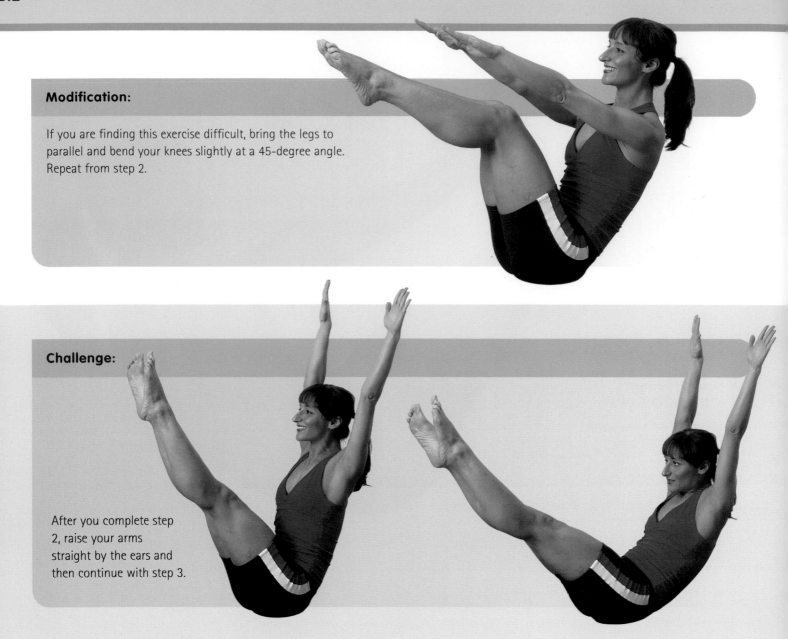

Modification:

If you are finding this exercise difficult, bring the legs to parallel and bend your knees slightly at a 45-degree angle. Repeat from step 2.

Challenge:

After you complete step 2, raise your arms straight by the ears and then continue with step 3.

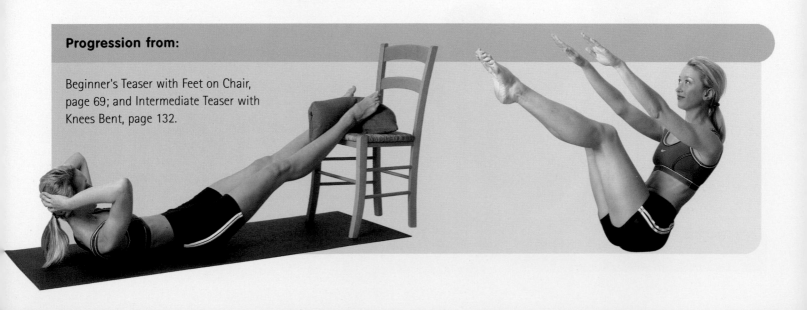

Progression from:

Beginner's Teaser with Feet on Chair, page 69; and Intermediate Teaser with Knees Bent, page 132.

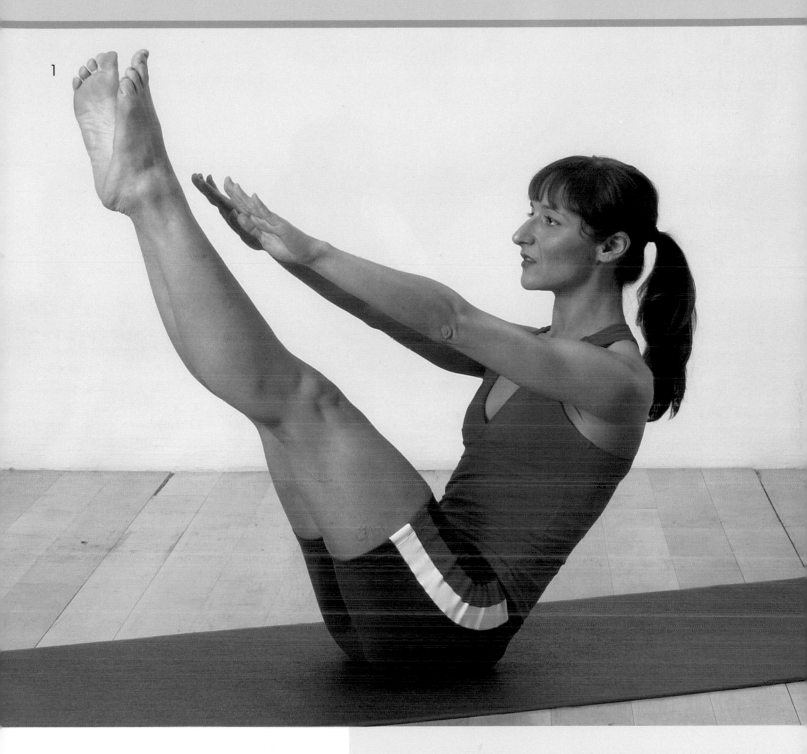

1

Teaser 2

The Teaser 2 works on balance and co-ordination, while focusing on strengthening the abdominals and inner thighs.

1 Start with your legs lifted high in the air at a 45-degree angle. Your toes should be apart and your heels together. Your upper torso is off the ground and your arms are reaching towards your feet. You are balancing slightly off your tailbone so the abdominals are engaged (Teaser position).

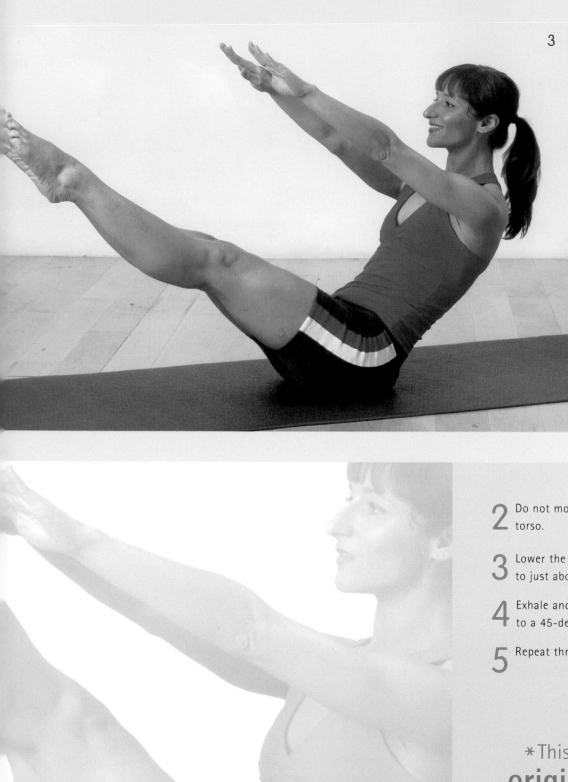

3

4

2 Do not move the upper torso.

3 Lower the legs as you inhale to just above the floor.

4 Exhale and lift the legs back to a 45-degree angle.

5 Repeat three to five times.

*This is an
original PILATES
*exercise**

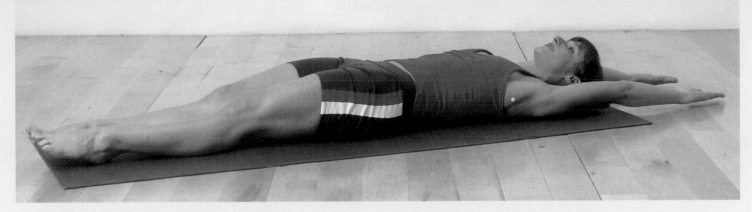

Transition: slowly lower the torso and legs down to the floor with the arms going over the head and the ribs in to prepare for Teaser 3.

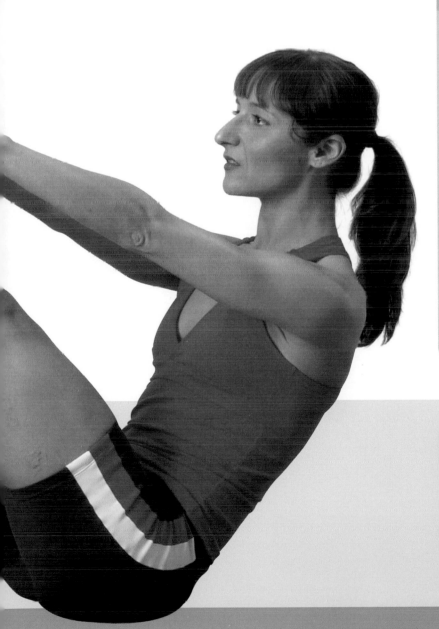

Key Points:

- If you have problems with your back, please leave this exercise out

- If your back starts to arch, please stop this exercise.

- Make sure the back rolls up and down sequentially.

- Keep the navel pulling into the spine and breathe through the back and sides of the ribs.

- Keep the shoulder blades pulling down the back.

- Lengthen through the toes and reach out through the fingertips.

- Glue the inner thighs together and squeeze the buttocks.

- Keep the upper torso still the whole time.

- Only lower the legs as low as you can control without losing stability.

- Do not arch! Do not let the arms whip!

Progression from: Teaser 2 on elbows, page 134.

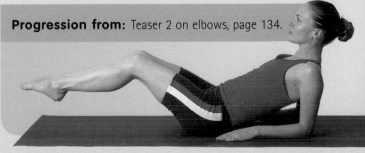

Teaser 3

The Teaser 3 incorporates all the principles of Pilates. It is a true test of strength, co-ordination and control.

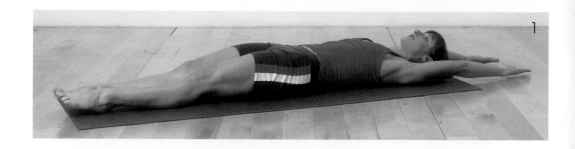

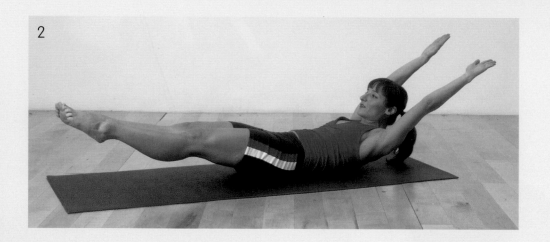

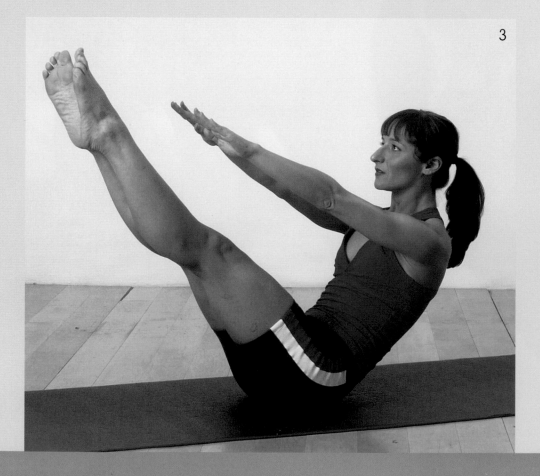

1 Lie on the ground with the legs and arms reaching in opposite directions. Your legs should be glued tight, with the toes apart and the heels together.

2 As you inhale, lift the arms and legs off the ground.

3 Roll all the way up to Teaser position.

4 Raise the arms by your ears.

5 Exhale and roll back down.

6 Repeat three times.

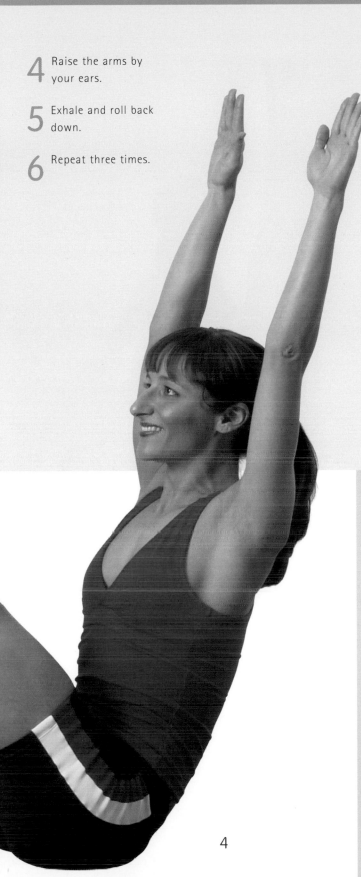

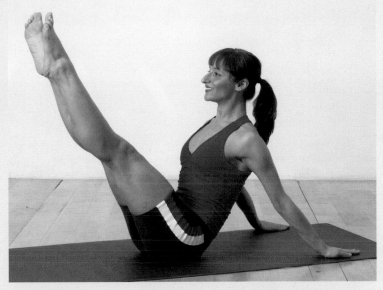

Transition: repeat one more movement and stop at the fourth step (Teaser position). Raise your arms by your ears and circle them down to the ground behind you. The fingertips are facing away from you with your chest open and your shoulders down. Ideally, try to bring your legs straight to the ceiling to prepare for Hip Circles.

Key Points:

- Make sure the back rolls up and down sequentially.

- Keep the navel pulling into the spine and breathe through the back and sides of the ribs.

- Keep the shoulder blades pulling down the back.

- Lengthen through the toes and reach out through the fingertips.

- Glue the inner thighs together and squeeze the buttocks.

- If your back starts to arch, please stop this exercise.

- Do not arch! Do not let the arms whip!

*This is an
original PILATES
exercise*

4

Hip Circles

This exercise strengthens the hips and stretches the legs, arms and chest while isolating the powerhouse.

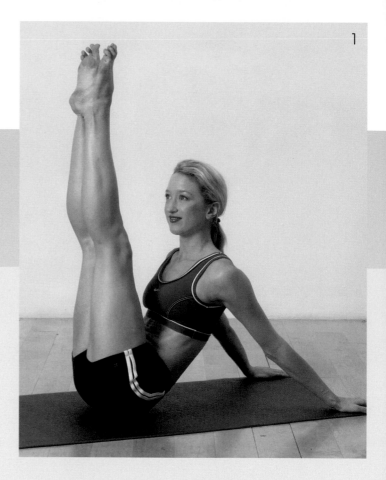

1 Sit up with your hands behind you, fingertips facing away. Your legs should be straight to the ceiling with heels together, toes apart. You are lifting up and out of your shoulders, while lengthening out of the hands and feet.

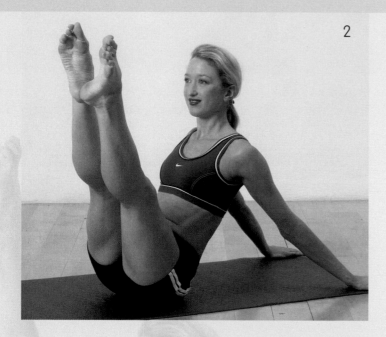

2 Inhale as you lower your legs down to the left.

3 Circle the legs around to the right and exhale as you lift the legs back to your nose.

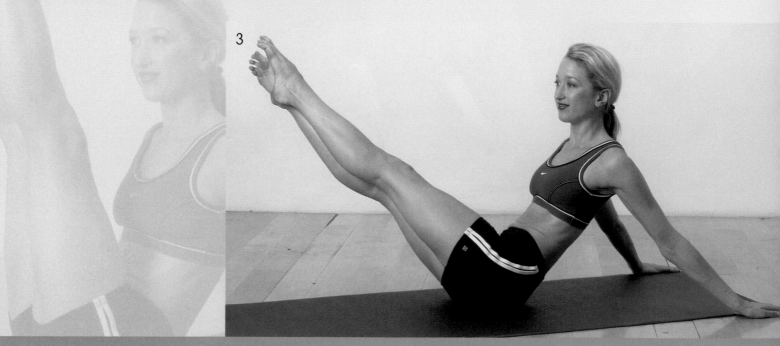

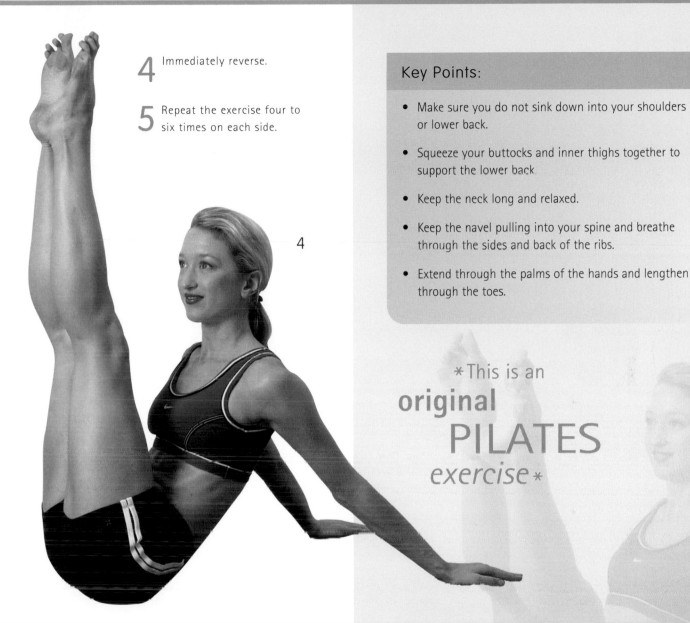

4 Immediately reverse.

5 Repeat the exercise four to six times on each side.

4

Key Points:

- Make sure you do not sink down into your shoulders or lower back.

- Squeeze your buttocks and inner thighs together to support the lower back.

- Keep the neck long and relaxed.

- Keep the navel pulling into your spine and breathe through the sides and back of the ribs.

- Extend through the palms of the hands and lengthen through the toes.

*This is an
original
PILATES
exercise

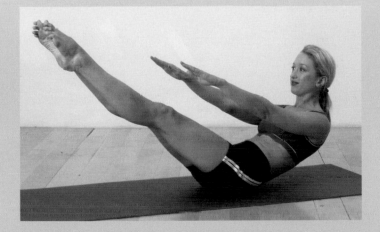

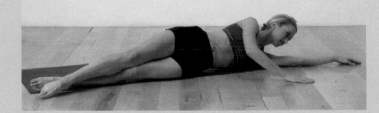

Transition: keeping the Teaser position, relax your hands towards your feet. Roll down through the spine as your legs lower and your arms reach overhead. Roll on to your stomach for Swimming.

Swimming

This exercise focuses on strengthening the muscles on either side of the spine while co-ordinating rhythm and control.

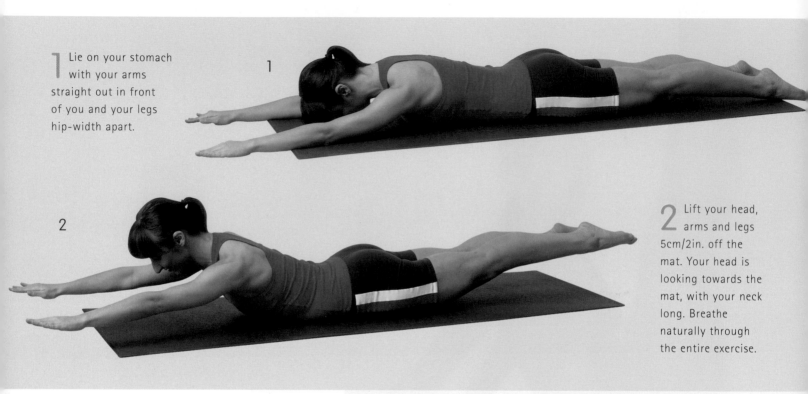

1 Lie on your stomach with your arms straight out in front of you and your legs hip-width apart.

2 Lift your head, arms and legs 5cm/2in. off the mat. Your head is looking towards the mat, with your neck long. Breathe naturally through the entire exercise.

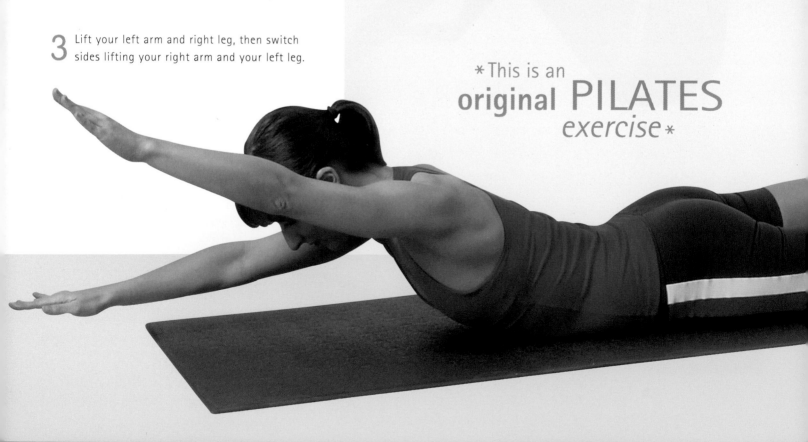

3 Lift your left arm and right leg, then switch sides lifting your right arm and your left leg.

*This is an
original PILATES
*exercise**

4 Quickly alternate arms and legs so that everything is moving in opposition without touching the floor.

5 Count to 20.

6 Relax.

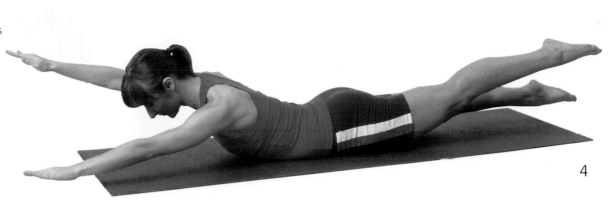

4

Transition: slide out into push-up position with your hands underneath your shoulders and your feet flexed back for Leg Pull-down.

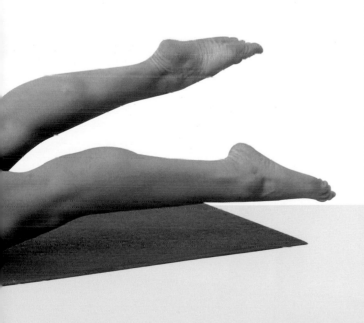

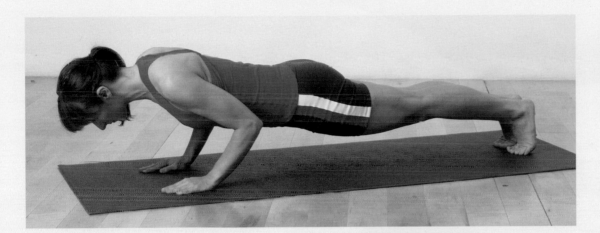

Key Points:

- Keep pulling your navel into your spine to support the lower back.
- Stretch your hands and feet in opposite directions.
- Keep your arms and legs straight.
- Do not bend the wrists.
- Do not crunch in the neck.

Progression from:

Shoulder Blades, page 55.

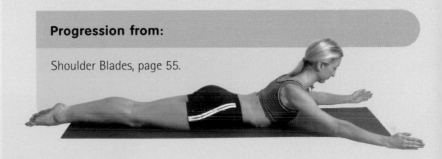

Leg Pull-down

The Leg Pull-down strengthens your shoulders, arms, abdominals, buttocks and hamstrings while stretching out your calves.

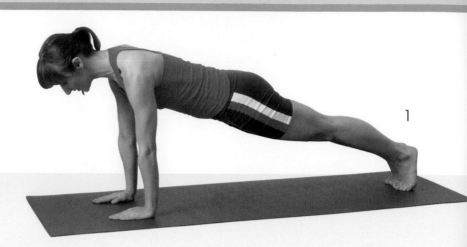

1

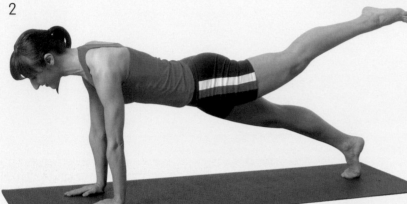

2

1 Start in full push-up position. Think of pressing your hands down through the floor underneath your shoulders. Your head is in line with your spine and your legs are extended behind you on your toes.

2 As you inhale, lift your left leg off the mat as high as you can without the hips coming out of alignment.

3 Hold your breath as you lower and lift the right ankle.

4 As you exhale, bring the left leg back to the original starting position.

5 As you take your next inhale, raise the right leg.

6 Hold your breath as you lower and lift the left ankle.

7 Exhale down.

8 Repeat three times each side.

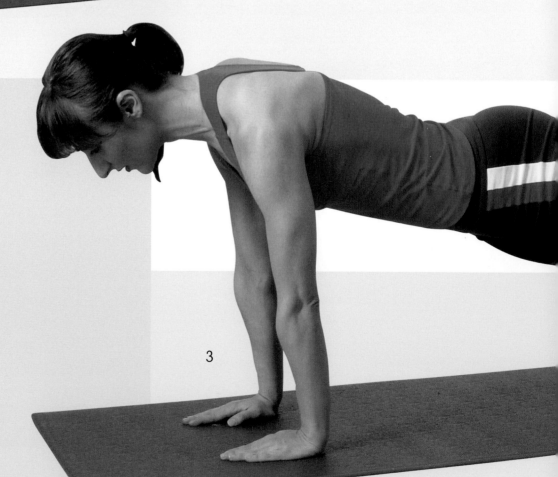

3

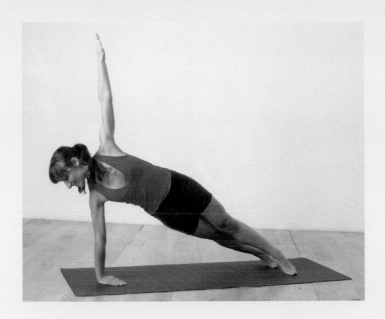

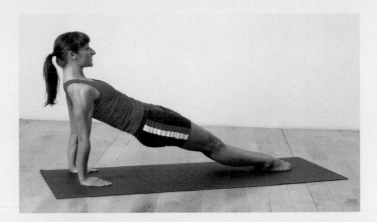

Transition: staying in push-up position, place the right hand next to the left. Slide fingers round to face toes. Flip the left arm high up and over to turn the whole body to face the ceiling. The pelvis should stay high for the Leg Pull-up.

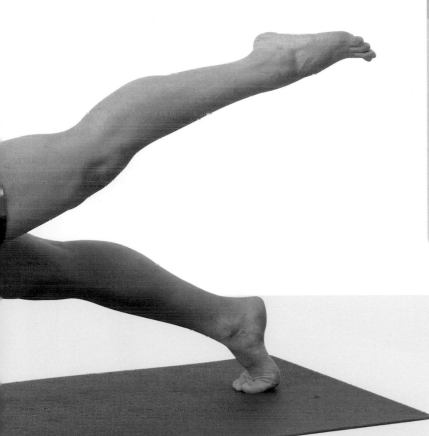

Key Points:

- Make sure your pelvis does not rock backwards as you lift the leg.

- Lengthen through the top of your head and out through the palms of your hands.

- Keep the navel pulling into your spine and breathe through the sides and back of your ribs.

- Make sure to stretch the calf every time you lower and lift the ankle.

- Do not arch your back.

*This is an
original
PILATES
exercise

Leg Pull-up

The Leg Pull-up strengthens your buttocks, shoulders and arms, while stretching your hamstrings.

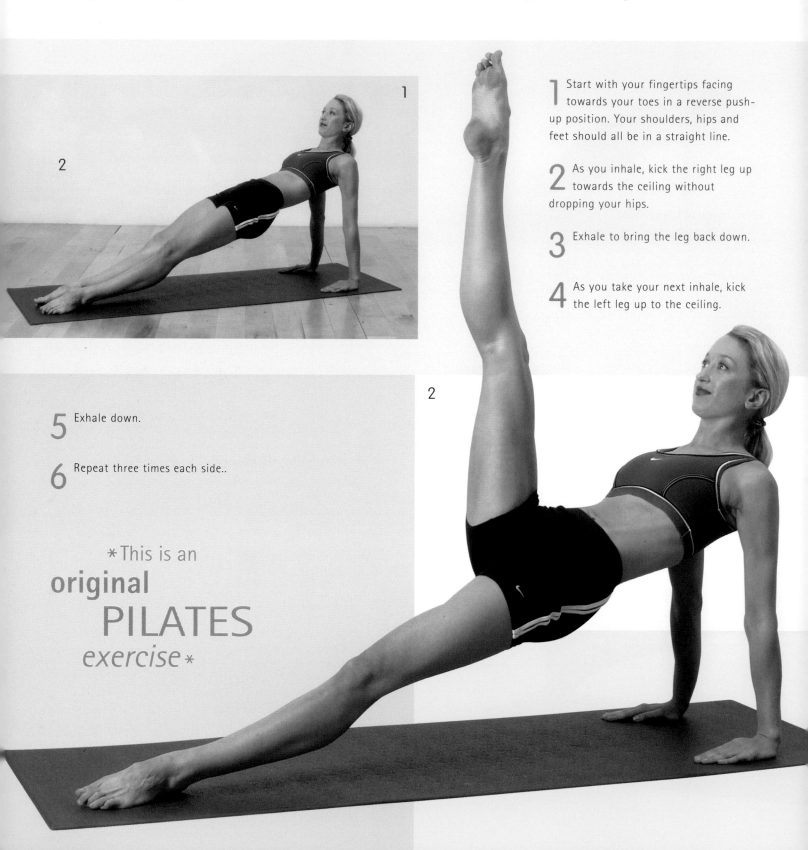

1   Start with your fingertips facing towards your toes in a reverse push-up position. Your shoulders, hips and feet should all be in a straight line.

2   As you inhale, kick the right leg up towards the ceiling without dropping your hips.

3   Exhale to bring the leg back down.

4   As you take your next inhale, kick the left leg up to the ceiling.

5   Exhale down.

6   Repeat three times each side..

*This is an
original
PILATES
exercise*

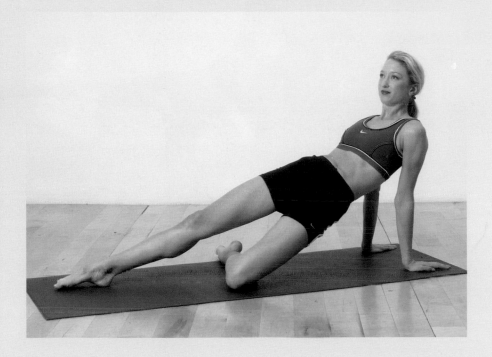

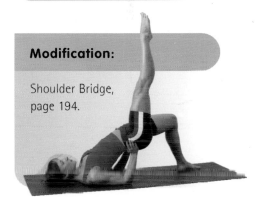

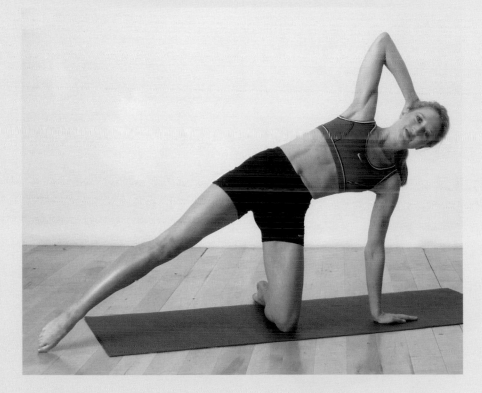

Transition: bend your left leg underneath you to face the left side of the mat. Your left hand stays on the ground as you place your right hand behind your head. Extend your right leg out along the mat and lift it up so that it is even with your hips for Side Kicks Kneeling.

Side Kicks Kneeling

This exercise focuses on balance, co-ordination and control. It strengthens the muscles of the waist, hips and legs.

1 Bend your right leg underneath you to face the right side of the mat. Your right hand stays on the ground as you place your left hand behind your head. Extend your left leg out along the mat and lift it up so that it is even with your hips.

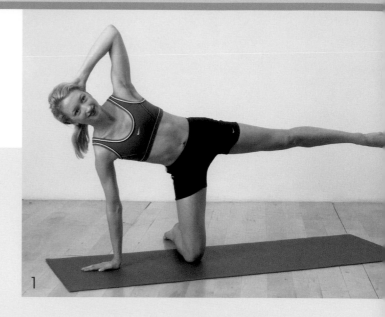

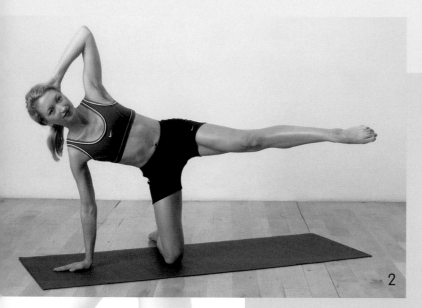

2 As you inhale, keep your upper torso quiet and kick the left leg in front of you twice, keeping the knee straight.

3 As you exhale, swing the left leg behind you and kick twice to the back.

4 Repeat five to eight times, then repeat on the other side.

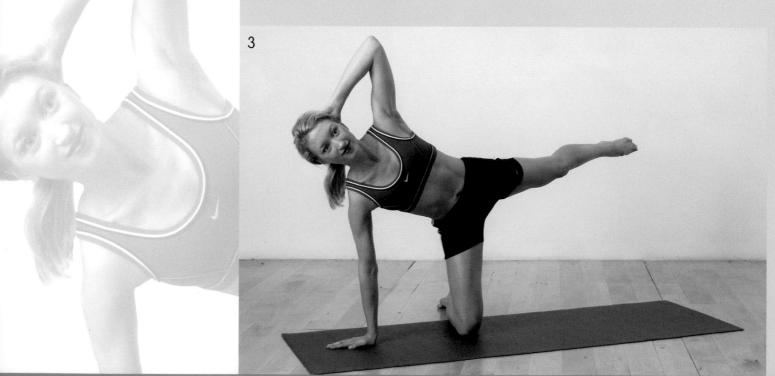

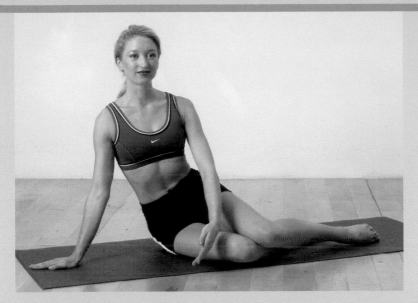

Transition: sit sideways, facing the right side of the mat. The left leg should be in front of the right, and the right arm straight. Your knees are bent and your left arm is rounded in front of your hips for the Twist.

Key Points:

- The upper body has a tendency to move during this exercise. Keep the torso as still as possible.

- Keep the leg long and the toes extending out through the space.

- Keep the elbow pointing towards the ceiling.

- Keep the navel pulling into the spine and breathe through the sides and back of the ribs.

- Keep the legs in parallel.

Challenge:

Once you have completed the kicking on one side, lift the right leg up 15cm/6in. towards the ceiling while pointing the ankle. Lower to hip height while flexing the ankle. Repeat five to eight times. Then circle the leg in one direction five times. Then reverse the circles five times. Repeat the whole sequence on the other side.

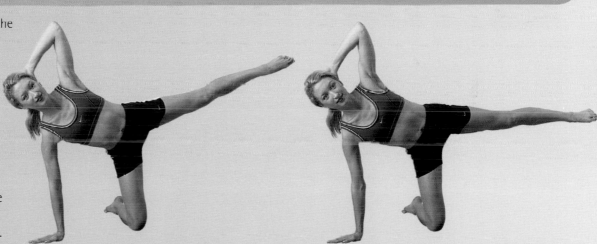

*This is an
original PILATES
exercise *

Modification:

Side Kicks, page 203.

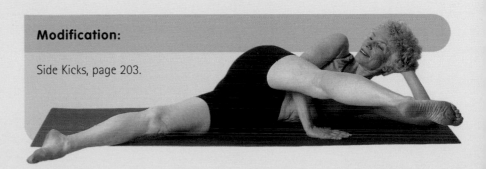

Twist

This exercise is designed for co-ordination, control, precision and flow of movement. Think of moving from your powerhouse.

1 Sit sideways, facing the right side. Your right hand is on the mat with your knees bent and your left leg slightly in front of the right. Your left arm is rounded down in front of your hips.

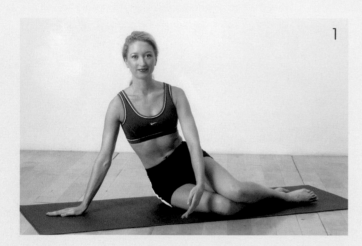

1

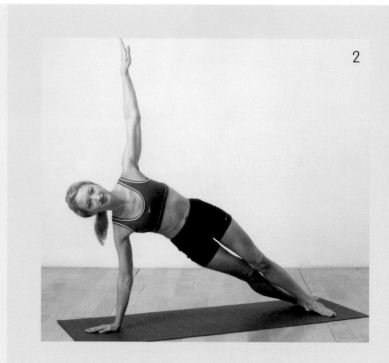

2

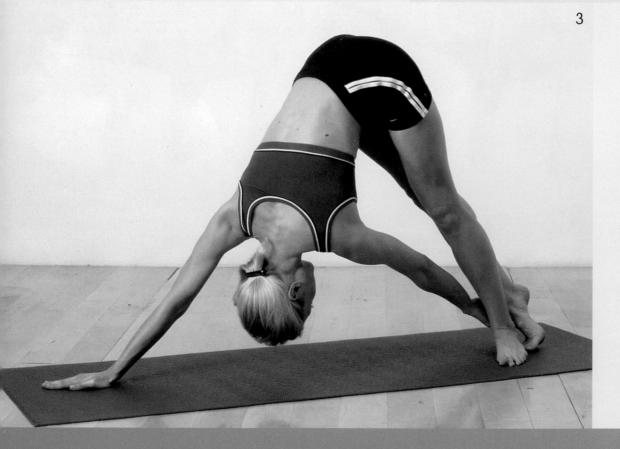

3

2 Inhale as you straighten your legs, lift your hips and extend your left hand towards the ceiling.

3 Exhale as you twist, reaching your left hand toward your right foot.

4

4 Inhale as you untwist, and lengthen your chest to the ceiling as your left arm reaches towards the left wall.

5 Exhale and relax back to a sitting position.

6 Repeat three times.

7 Repeat on the other side.

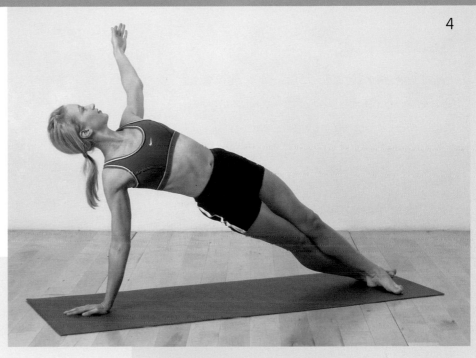

Transition: sit down on your mat with your right foot crossed over the left and your hands by your sides for the Boomerang.

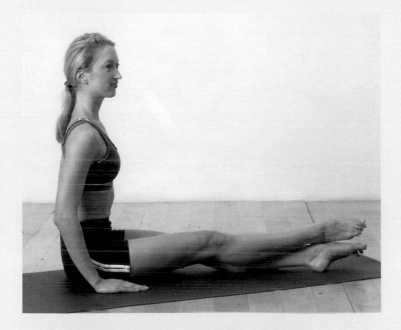

Key Points:

- Make sure you are moving from the abdominals.

- Press out through the hands.

- Keep the navel pulling into your spine and breathe through the sides and back of your ribs.

- Do not sink into your shoulders.

Challenge:

Once you have mastered this exercise, try stacking your feet one on top of the other.

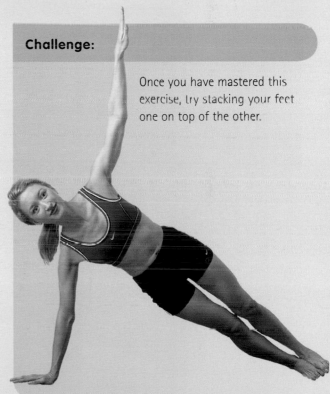

*This is an
original PILATES
exercise

Boomerang

The Boomerang is one of the most advanced exercises in Pilates. Focus on controlling the movement from the powerhouse.

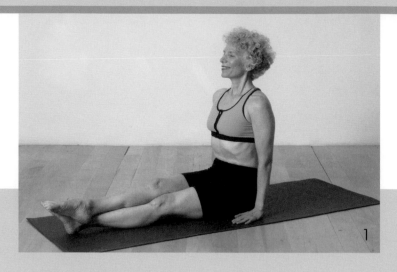

1 Sit up with your legs straight and cross your right ankle over your left. Place one hand on either side of your hips.

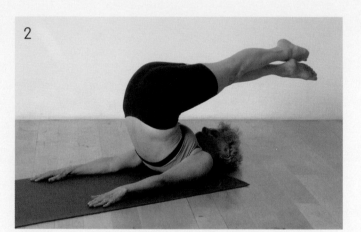

2 As you inhale, roll backwards from the powerhouse in one piece. You want your legs to be parallel over your head behind you.

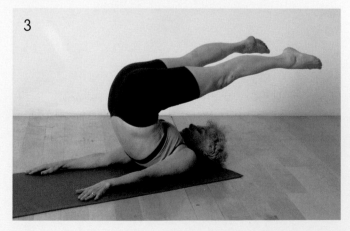

3 As you exhale, stay where you are and quickly open and close your legs . . .

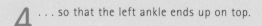

4 . . . so that the left ankle ends up on top.

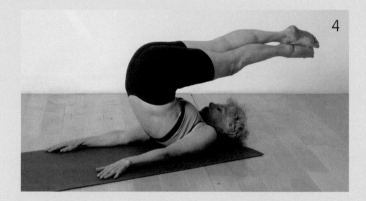

5 Inhale as you roll all the way back up so that you end up in Teaser position with your legs crossed. Your hands should be reaching towards your ankles.

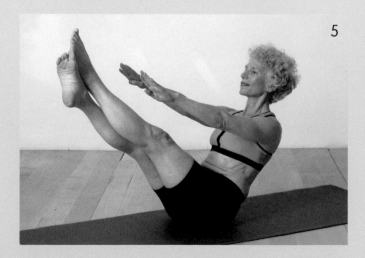

6

6 Turn the hands over so the palms are facing the ceiling. Bring your elbows back behind you and clasp your hands.

7 Exhale as you lift the arms up and bring your legs to the floor, trying to touch your nose to your knee. Unclasp the hands and circle them around to your feet

8 Stretch the hamstrings and prepare to start again.

9 Repeat three times.

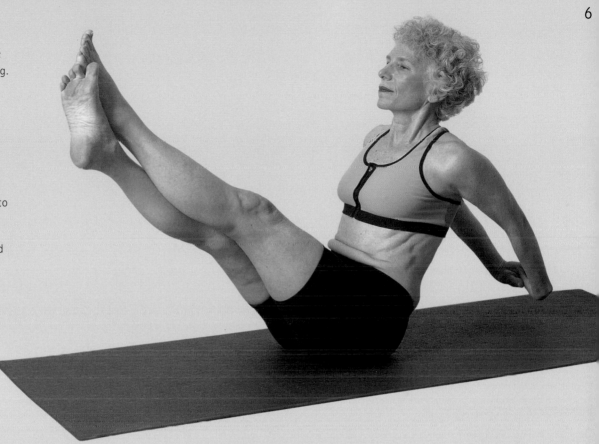

Transition: bend your knees and place the soles of the feet together. Circle your arms through the hoop and hold on to your ankles. Lift your feet off the floor for Seal.

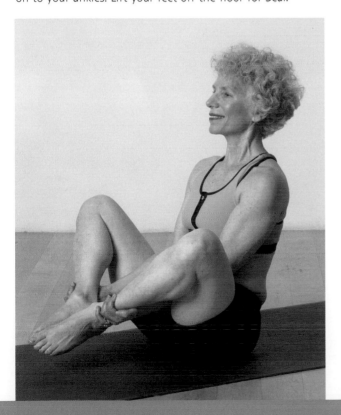

Key Points:

- Focus on trying to lift everything down to the floor in one piece.

- Keep the legs straight.

- Move the torso and legs in one piece.

- Straighten your arms in Teaser position before lowering your legs.

- Keep the navel pulling into your spine and breathe through the sides and back of the ribs.

*This is an
original PILATES
exercise *

Seal

The Seal is a great exercise after the Boomerang. Think of rounding the back while focusing on control.

1 Sit up with the soles of the feet together and the knees out to the sides. Place your hands under your lower calves and hold on to your ankles. Lift the feet off the ground and balance on your tailbone.

2 Clap the feet together three times.

*This is an **original** PILATES *exercise**

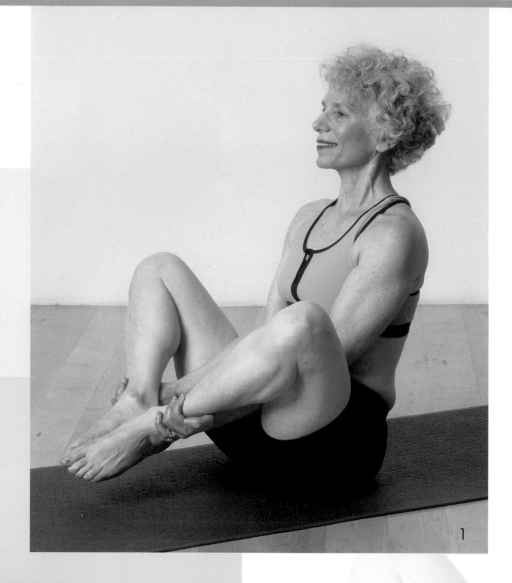

1

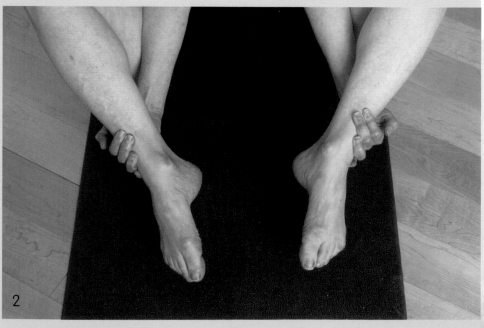

2

3 Inhale rolling backwards so the feet are 30cm/12in. off the ground behind you. Clap the feet together three times.

4 Exhale and roll back up.

5 Repeat four to eight times.

3

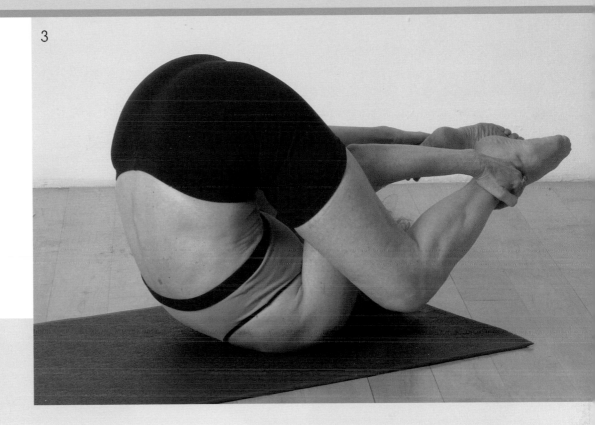

Transition: cross the legs and hold on to your feet with your hands for the Crab.

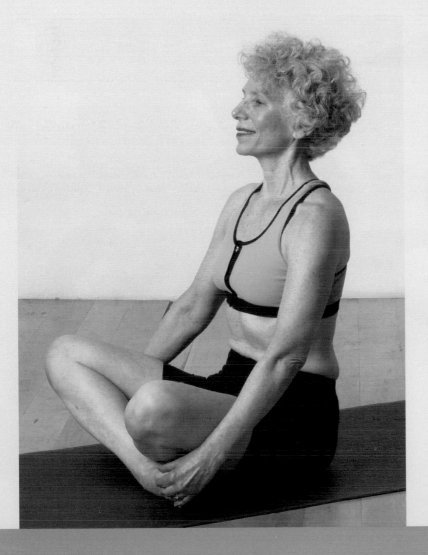

Key Points:

- Clap with the whole leg, not just the feet.
- Keep the shoulder blades pulling down the back
- Keep the navel pulling into the spine and breathe through the sides and back of the ribs.
- Do not let the head go out as you roll backwards.
- Do not go crashing back on to your neck. Roll back to the top of your shoulders.

Modification:

Rolling Like A Ball, page 154.

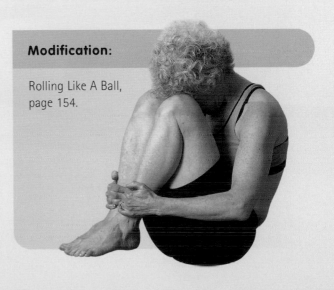

Crab

The Crab focuses on control and co-ordination from the powerhouse. It is also good for getting rid of headaches!

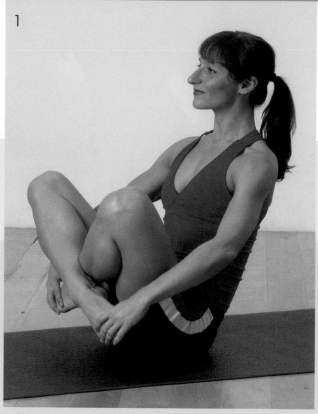

1 Start with your knees bent and crossed, one leg over the other. Hold on to the feet with your hands. Lift your feet off the mat.

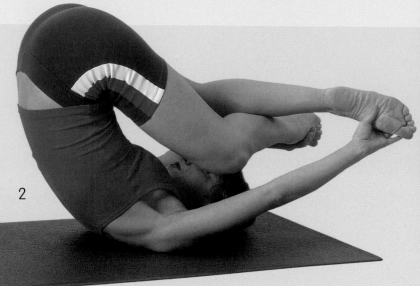

2 Inhale and control from the abdominals as you roll backwards in one piece on to the shoulders.

3 Hold your breath as you let go of the feet and change so that the other leg is crossed in front.

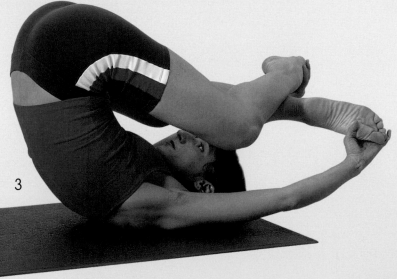

4 Grab the feet as you exhale and lean forwards, rolling on to the forehead with the buttocks in the air.

5 Slowly sit back on your pelvis to start again.

6 Repeat four to eight times.

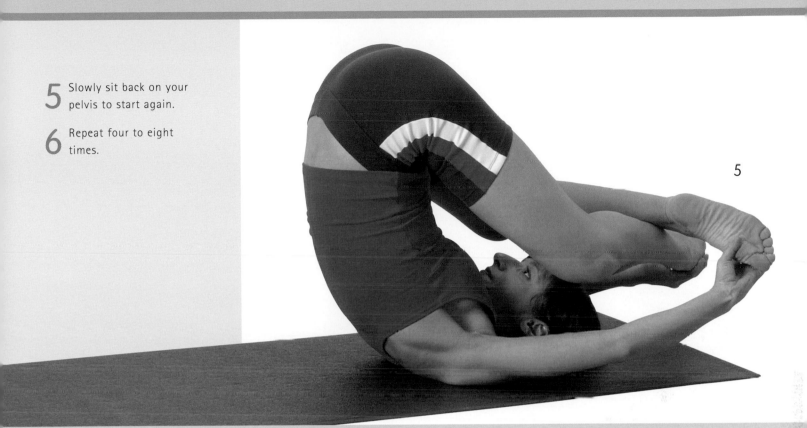

5

Transition: let go of your feet and turn over on to your stomach for the Rocking.

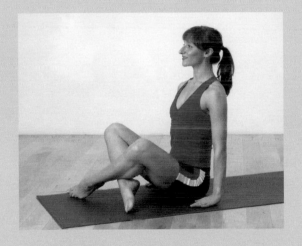

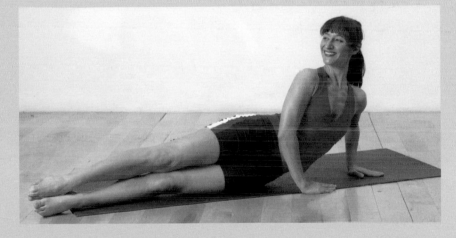

Key Points:

• Keep the shoulder blades pulling down the back.

• Keep the navel pulling into your spine and breathe through the sides and back of the ribs.

• Do not crash on to the head! Slowly roll up on to the top of the head.

*This is an
original
PILATES
exercise *

Rocking

The Rocking is a great stretch for your shoulders, chest, back and quadriceps.

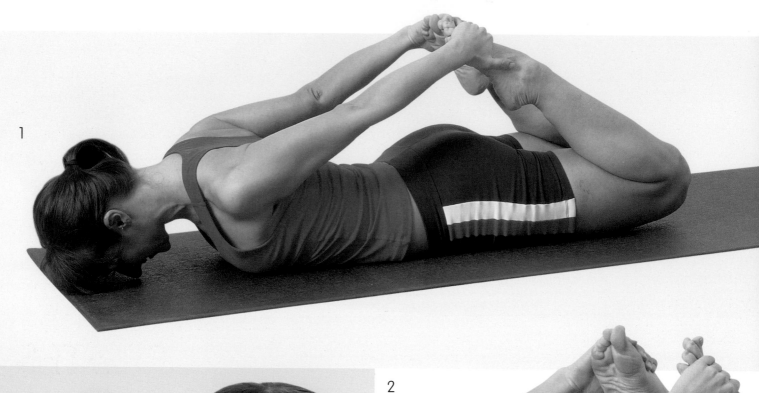

1

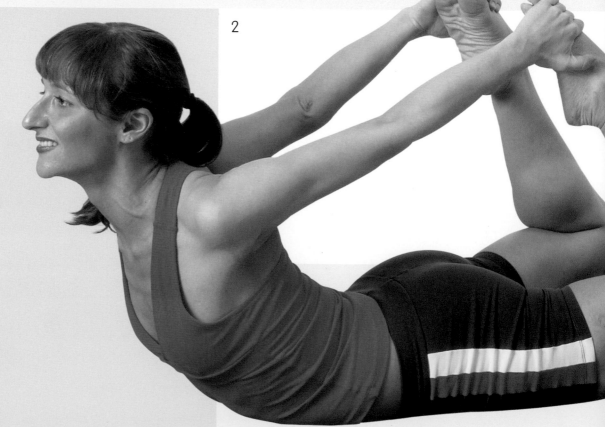

2

1 Lie on your stomach with your knees bent. Hold on to your feet behind you, one foot in each hand. Bring your knees as close together as possible.

2 As you inhale, pull your navel into your spine and stretch your hands and feet up to the ceiling.

3 Exhale to relax down.

4 Repeat one more time.

5 On the next lift up, stay there. Thinking of moving from your abdominals, rock slowly towards your shoulders and inhale, then slowly back towards your hips and exhale.

6 Relax.

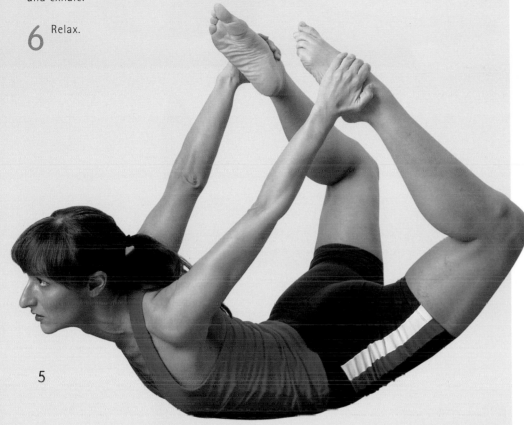

5

Key Points:

- Please leave this exercise out if you have problems with your back.

- Keep your knees as close together as possible.

- Rock from the abdominals, not the head or legs.

- Keep the navel pulling into your ribs and breathe through the sides and back of the ribs.

* This is an
original
PILATES
exercise *

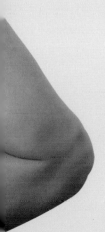

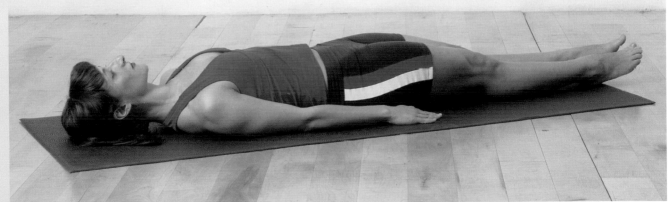

Transition: lie out long and roll over on to your back for the Control Balance.

Control Balance

The Control Balance focuses on exactly that – control! It stretches the spine, shoulders and hamstrings while strengthening the buttocks and abdominals.

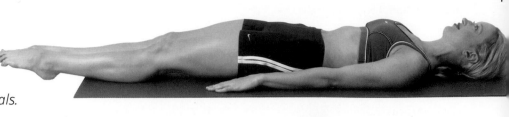

1

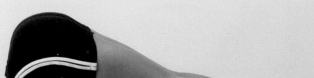

2

1 Lie on your back with your legs out straight along the mat and your arms down by your sides.

2 Pull your navel into your spine and lift your legs off the ground.

3 Roll up on to your shoulders and place the feet on the mat behind you with straight legs.

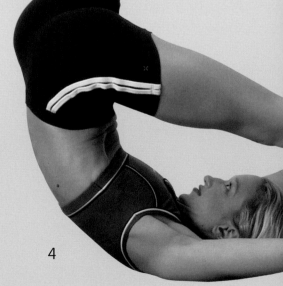

3

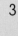

4

4 Reach both hands over your head and hold on to your left ankle. Extend your right leg towards the ceiling.

5 Controlling the movement from the abdominals and buttocks, change the legs, letting them pass each other in the air.

6 Inhale as the legs switch, and exhale on the ends.

7 Repeat four times.

5

* This is an
original
PILATES
exercise *

Transition: as you roll down sequentially through the spine, cross the ankles and the arms and stand straight up. Walk to the back of the mat for the Push-ups.

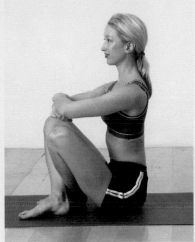

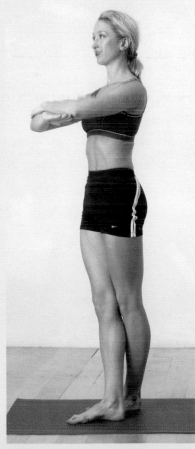

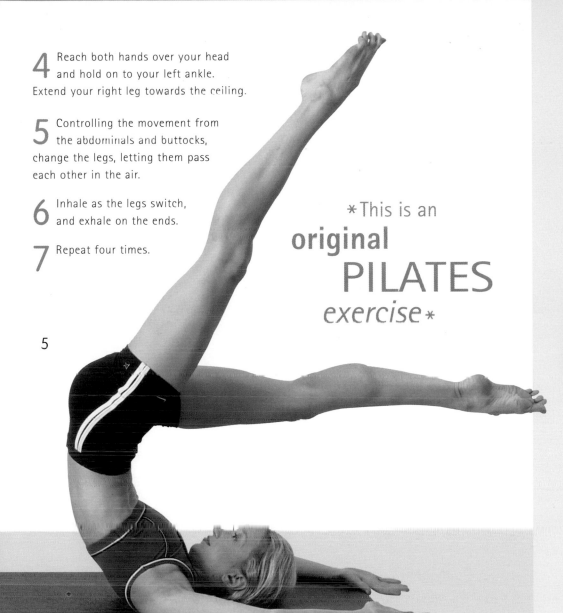

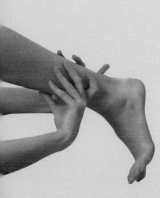

Key Points:

- Extend through the toes.

- Keep the legs straight.

- Keep the navel pulling into your spine and breathe through the sides and back of the ribs.

- Do not go up on to the neck. Make sure your weight is on the shoulders and you are controlling the movement from the abdominals and buttocks.

Push-ups

This exercise strengthens the shoulders, abdominals and arms, while stretching the back and hamstrings.

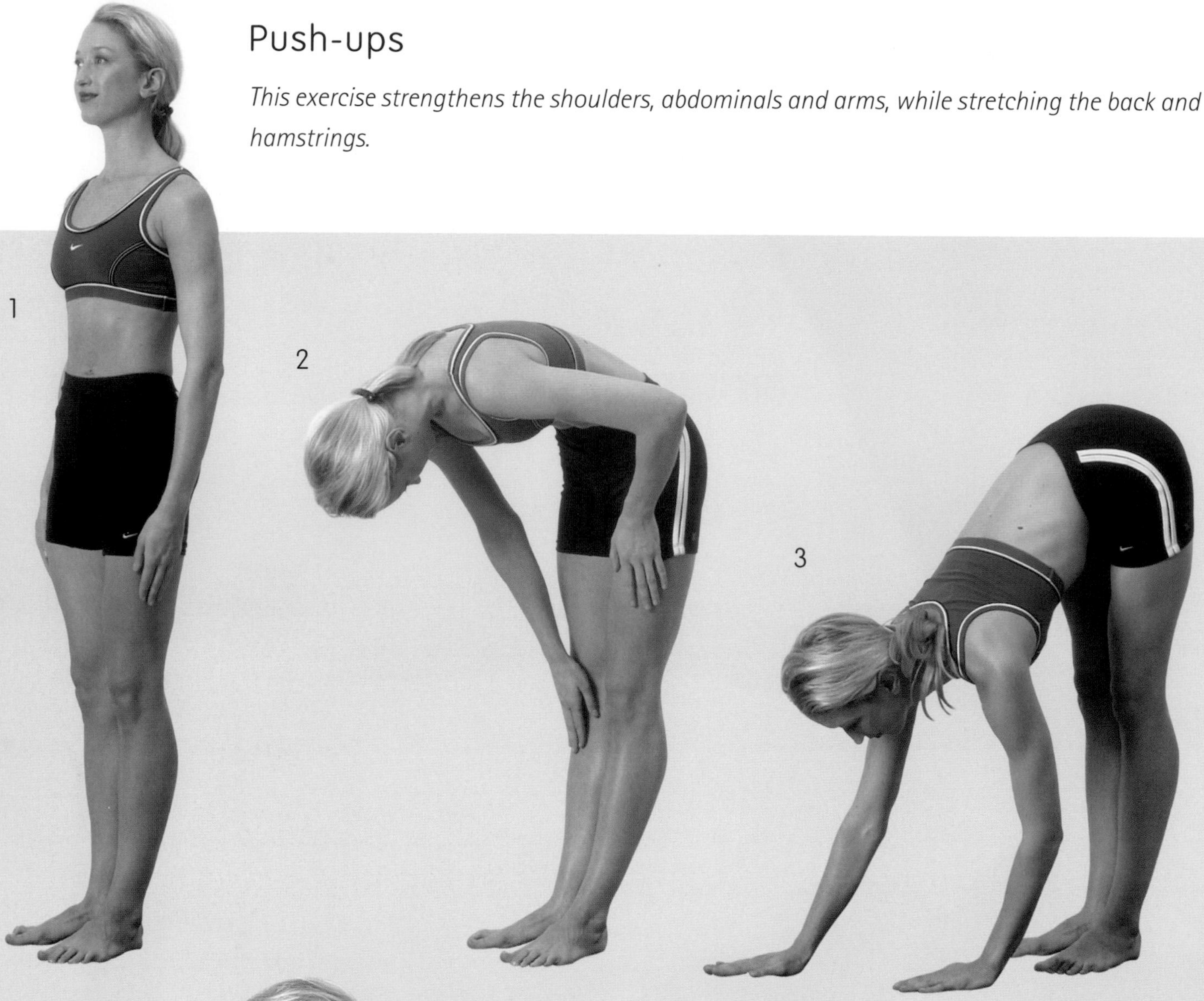

1

2

3

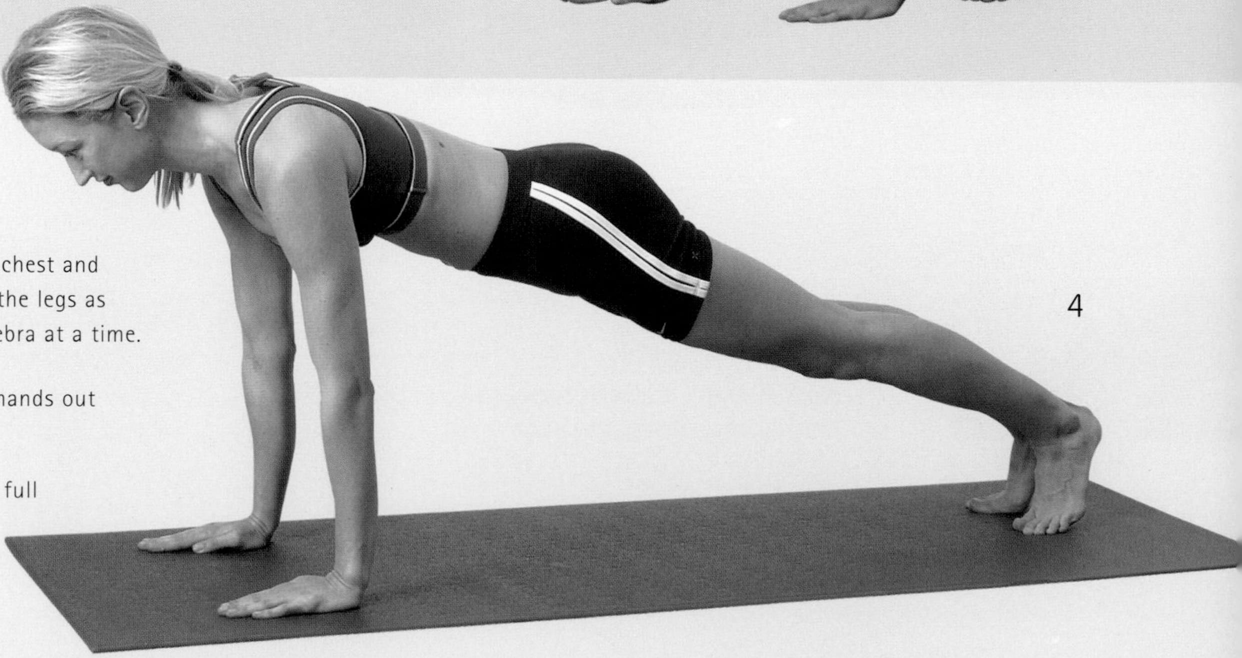

1 Stand up facing
your mat.

2 Curl the chin into the chest and
walk the hands down the legs as
you roll forwards one vertebra at a time.

3 Continue to walk the hands out
along the mat . . .

4 . . . until you are in a full
push-up position.

4

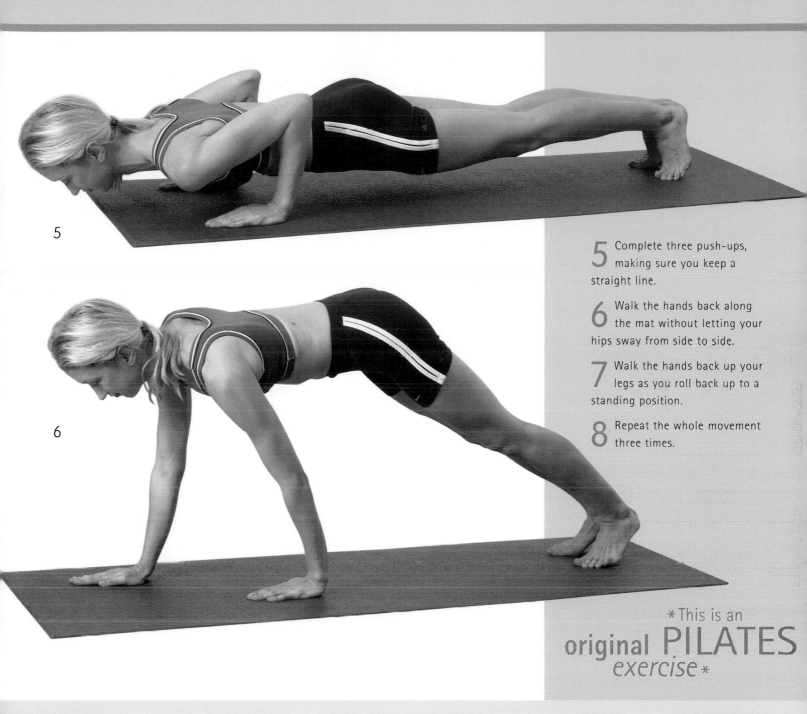

5

6

5 Complete three push-ups, making sure you keep a straight line.

6 Walk the hands back along the mat without letting your hips sway from side to side.

7 Walk the hands back up your legs as you roll back up to a standing position.

8 Repeat the whole movement three times.

*This is an
original PILATES
exercise*

Key Points:

- Keep the hips square.

- Keep the shoulder blades pulling down the back.

- Do not let the hips sway from side to side as you walk the hands out along the mat and back again.

- Make sure you do not arch on the push-ups. Only go as low as you can control.

Progression from:

Triceps push-ups, page 122.

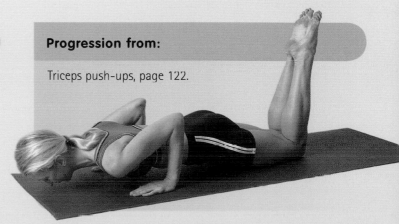

Arm series

The arm series in Pilates is usually performed at the end of a session. The weights are lighter than those used in a typical gym work-out. The objective is to tone without building bulk. Women should use weights no heavier than 2kg, while men's weights should be no more than 3kg.

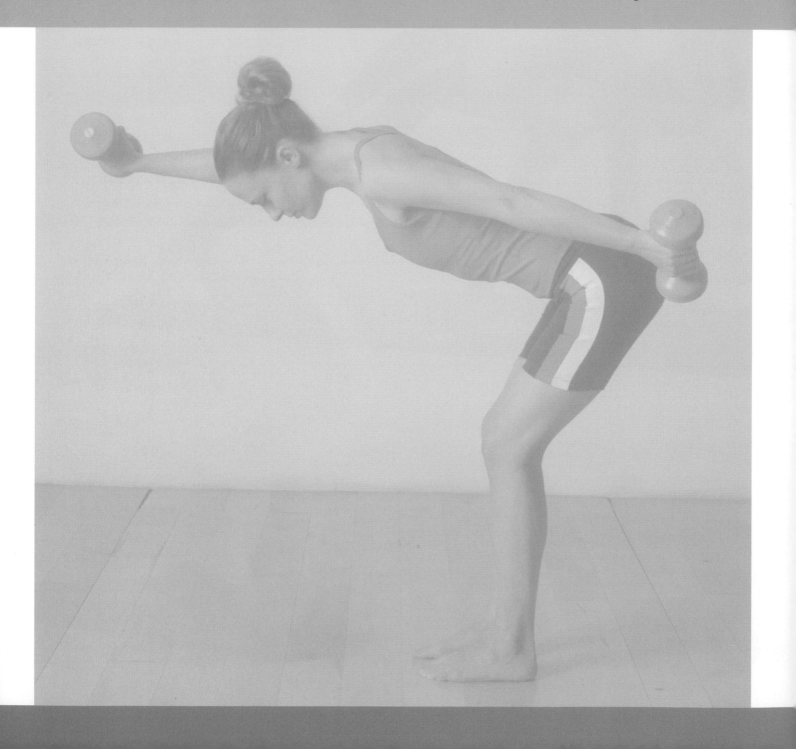

Arms 1

This exercise works the biceps, deltoids and chest muscles (pectoralis major).

You will need: small weights, 2kg for women, 3kg for men.

1 Stand with one weight in each hand. Place your toes apart and your heels together. Lengthen your head towards the ceiling.

2 Pull your navel into your spine and bring your hands towards your shoulders. Lift your elbows up so that they are parallel to the ground and each other. Inhale to prepare.

3 As you exhale, extend the arms straight out in front of you.

4 Inhale and think of pressing against a very heavy weight as you bring the hands back towards the shoulders.

5 Repeat the whole exercise ten times.

Key Points:

- Make sure the lower back is relaxed. If it feels tense, you might want to lean against a wall.

- Keep the shoulder blades pulling down the back.

- Keep the inner thighs and buttocks squeezed tight together.

- Extend through the top of your head and lengthen down through the floor.

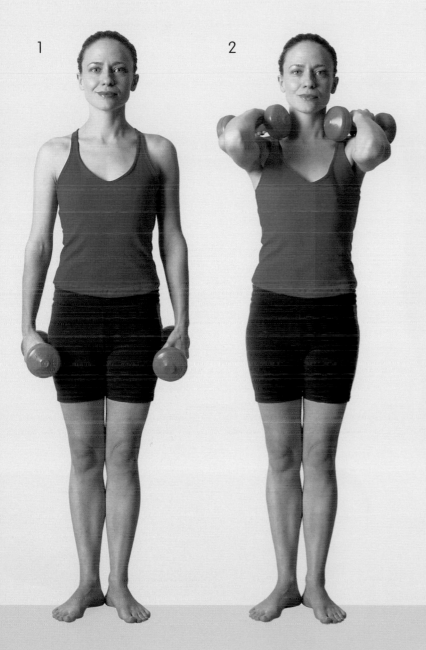

1

2

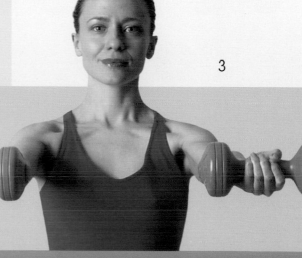

3

*This is an
original PILATES
exercise *

Arms 2

This exercise works the biceps and deltoids.

You will need: small weights.

1 Stay in the same position as exercise 1, but slightly move your elbows to the sides so that they are in a diagonal in front of you. Inhale to prepare.

2 Lift your elbows, bringing weights to your shoulders.

3 Exhale to extend, keeping the biceps parallel to the floor.

4 Repeat ten times.

Key Points:

- Make sure the lower back is relaxed. If it feels tense, you might want to lean against a wall.

- Keep the shoulder blades pulling down the back.

- Keep the inner thighs and buttocks squeezed tight together.

- Extend through the top of your head and lengthen down through the floor.

- Make sure the elbows stay slightly forwards so that you do not put too much pressure on the shoulder cuff.

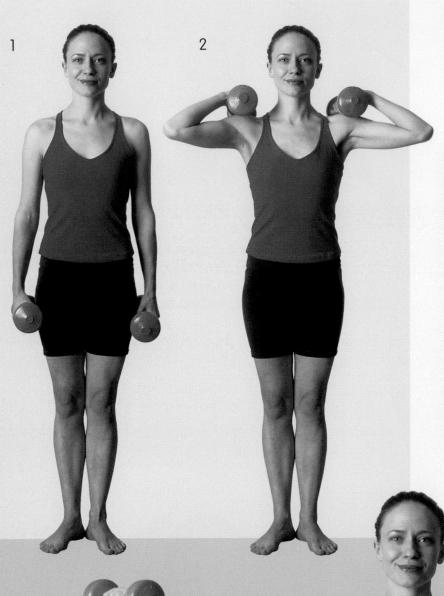

*This is an
original PILATES
exercise*

Arms 3

This exercise focuses on the triceps.

You will need: small weights.

1 Start with one weight in each hand. Stand with your feet hip-width apart and parallel to each other. Bend your knees and bring your upper torso forwards so that you have a flat back like a table top. Your upper torso should be parallel to the floor. Bend your elbows to the ceiling. Ideally, your elbows should be higher than your torso and parallel to each other. Inhale to prepare.

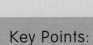

2 As you exhale, keep the elbows where they are and extend your forearms towards the ceiling behind you. Inhale back to your original position.

3 Repeat ten times.

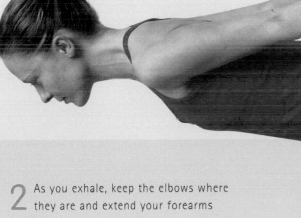

This is an
original
 PILATES
exercise *

Key Points:

• Keep the navel pulling into your spine and breathe through the sides and back of the ribs.

• Lengthen out through the top of your head.

• Keep the knees bent and parallel to each other.

• Do not put pressure on your lower back! Keep the lower back long.

Arms 4

This exercise focuses on the shoulders and arms.

You will need: small weights.

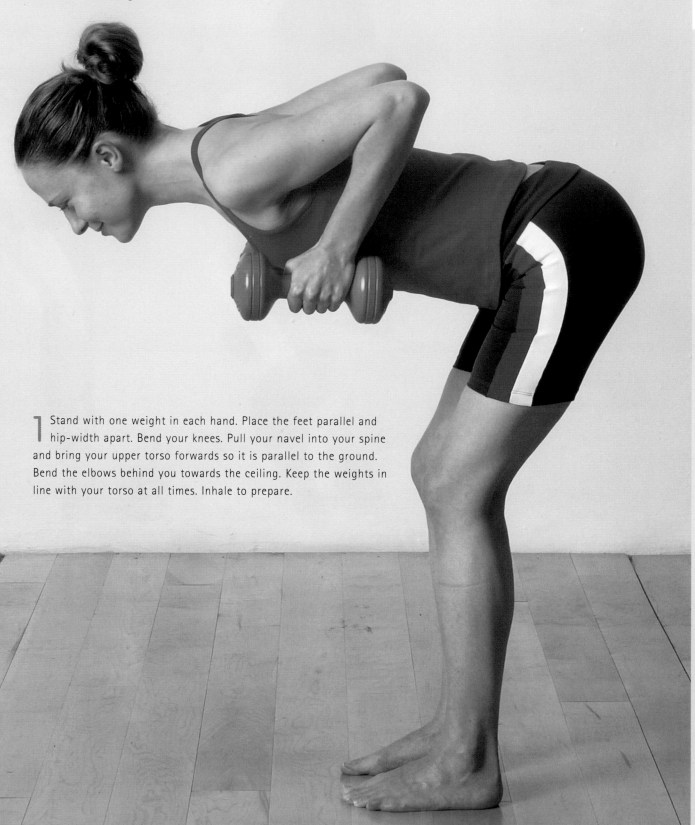

1 Stand with one weight in each hand. Place the feet parallel and hip-width apart. Bend your knees. Pull your navel into your spine and bring your upper torso forwards so it is parallel to the ground. Bend the elbows behind you towards the ceiling. Keep the weights in line with your torso at all times. Inhale to prepare.

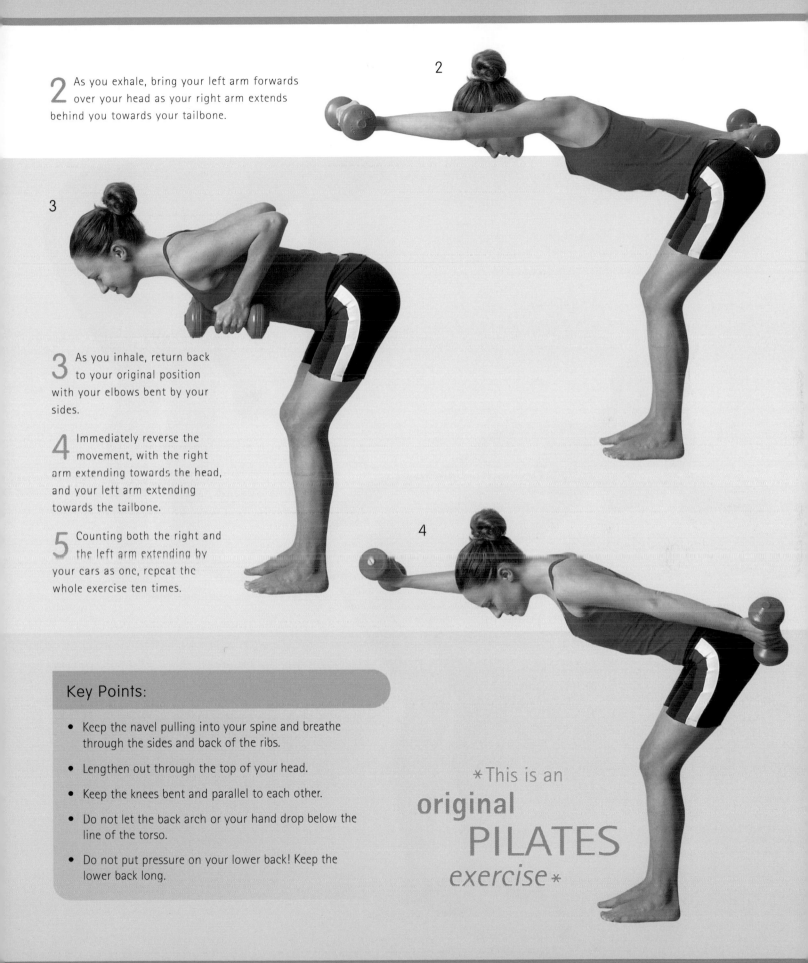

2 As you exhale, bring your left arm forwards over your head as your right arm extends behind you towards your tailbone.

2

3

3 As you inhale, return back to your original position with your elbows bent by your sides.

4 Immediately reverse the movement, with the right arm extending towards the head, and your left arm extending towards the tailbone.

5 Counting both the right and the left arm extending by your ears as one, repeat the whole exercise ten times.

4

Key Points:

- Keep the navel pulling into your spine and breathe through the sides and back of the ribs.

- Lengthen out through the top of your head.

- Keep the knees bent and parallel to each other.

- Do not let the back arch or your hand drop below the line of the torso.

- Do not put pressure on your lower back! Keep the lower back long.

*This is an
original
PILATES
exercise*

Arms 5

This exercise focuses on the muscles around your shoulder blades, the rhomboids and trapezius.

You will need: small weights.

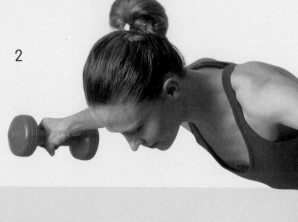

1 Stand and place one weight in each hand. The feet should be hip-width apart and parallel to each other. Bend your knees. Bring your upper torso forwards so that it is parallel to the ground and the back is flat like a table top. Make a circle with your arms towards the floor. Pull your navel into your spine. Inhale to prepare.

2 Keeping your elbows at the same angle, exhale and bring your shoulder blades together while raising your arms to the sides.

3 Inhale and return the arms to the original position.

4 Repeat the whole movement ten times.

This is an **original** **PILATES** *exercise*

Key Points:

- Keep the navel pulling into your spine and breathe through the sides and back of the ribs.

- Lengthen out through the top of your head.

- Keep the knees bent and parallel to each other.

- Do not arch your back while pulling your shoulder blades together.

- Do not put pressure on your lower back! Keep the lower back long.

Arms 6

This exercise focuses on the triceps.

You will need: small weights.

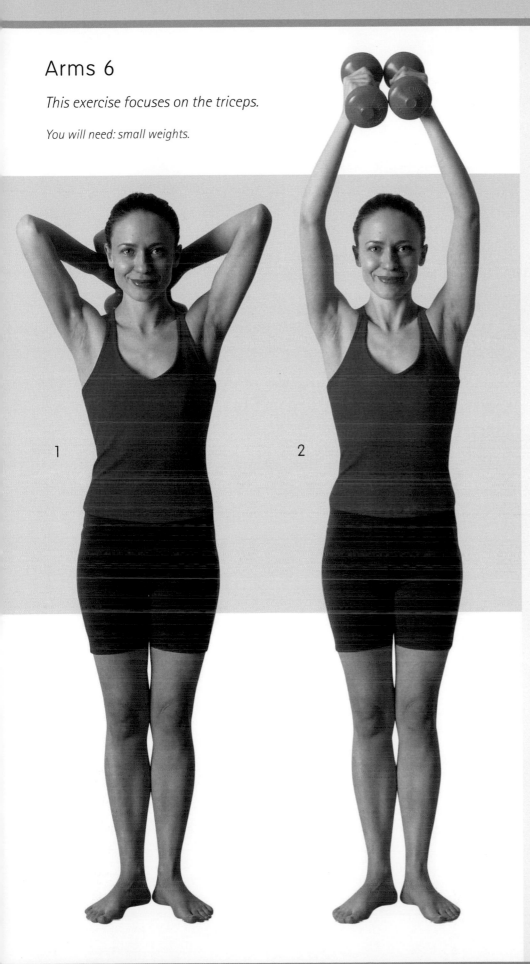

1

2

1 Stand with one weight in each hand, with toes apart, heels together. Place the hands with the weights touching behind the nape of the neck and the elbows to the sides. Make sure the head is in line with the spine and you are not looking at the floor. Inhale to prepare.

2 As you exhale, extend the hands towards the ceiling.

3 Inhale to relax the hands back behind the nape of the neck.

4 Repeat ten times.

Key Points:

- Keep the shoulder blades pulling down the back.

- Keep the inner thighs and buttocks squeezed tight together.

- Extend through the top of your head and lengthen down through the floor.

- Do not let the back arch.

*This is an **original PILATES** *exercise**

Advanced 15-minute workout

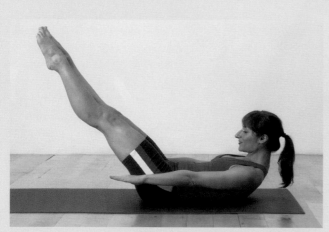

Hundred page 144.

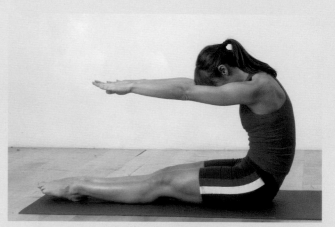

Roll-up page 145.

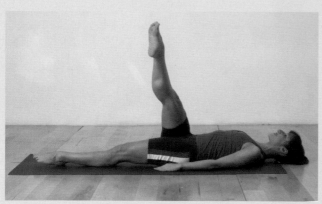

Leg Circles page 151.

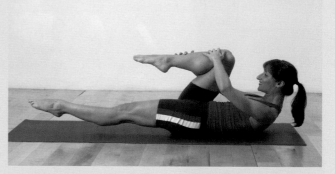

Single Leg Stretch page 156.

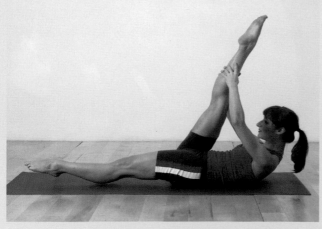

Single Straight Leg Stretch page 160.

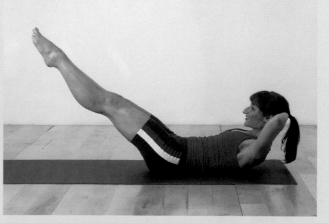

Single Straight Leg Stretch page 162.

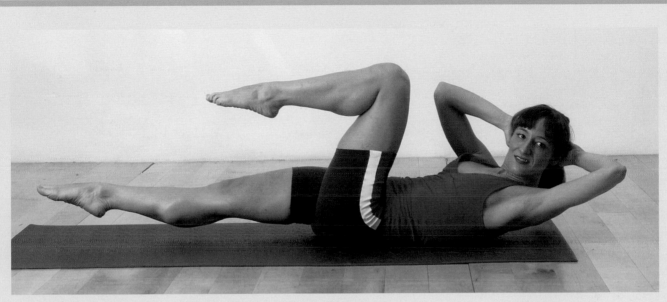

Criss Cross page 164.

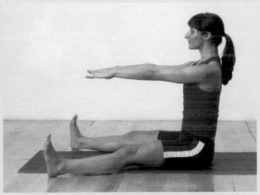

Spine Stretch Forward page 166.

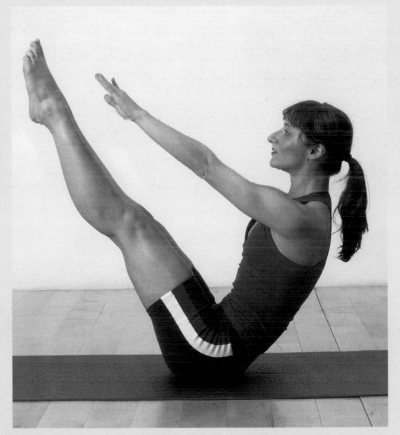

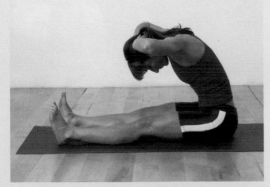

Neck Pull 186.

Teaser 1 page 210.

General Terms

Abdominals This generally means the rectus abdominals, unless otherwise stated.

Biceps The muscle on the front of the upper arm.

Buttocks The gluteus minimus, medius and maximus.

Extension To stretch or lengthen out.

Flexion Bending or curling.

Hamstrings The three muscles on the back of the thigh.

Inner thighs The adductors and gracilis.

Navel to spine Pulling the bellybutton back towards your spine.

Neck exercises Either stretching or strengthening the back and sides of the neck.

Quadriceps The four muscles on the front of the thigh.

Triceps The muscle in the back of the upper arm.

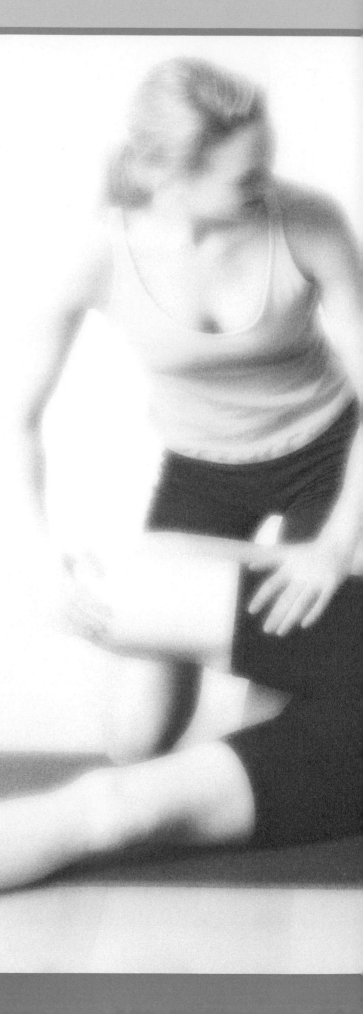

Bibliography

Friedman, Philip

The Pilates Method of Physical and Mental Conditioning

(Studio Books 1980)

Pilates, Joseph *(Ed.)*

The Pilates Return to Life through Contrology

(Presentation Dynamics Inc, 1998)

Selby, Anne

Pilates Creating the Body you Want

(Gaia Books Ltd, 1999)

Siler, Brook

The Pilates Body

(Penguin Books Ltd, 2000)

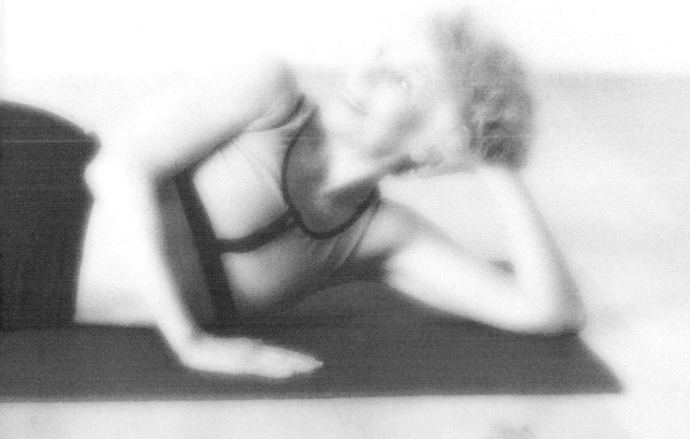

Index

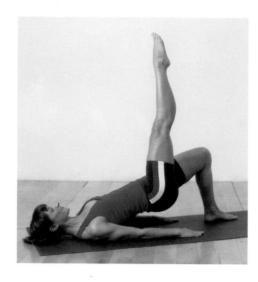

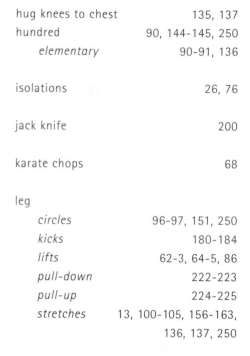

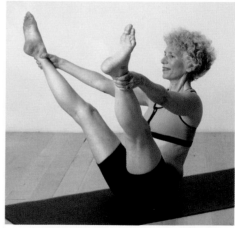

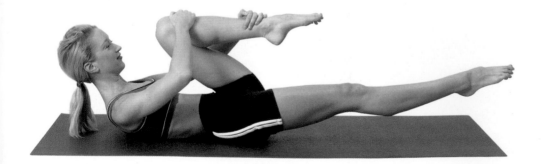

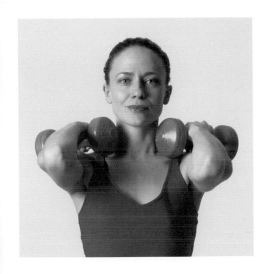

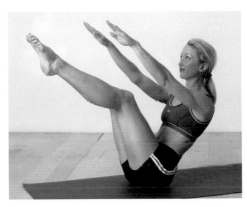

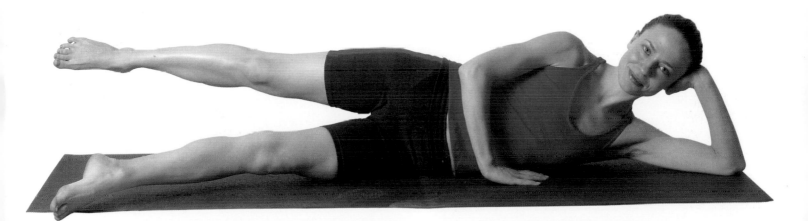

Credits and acknowledgements

Key Consultants

I owe much thanks to the contributions and endless advice from:

Phoebe Higgins

Phoebe Higgins began studying Pilates in 1976 with Romana Kryzanowska at SUNY at Purchase. In 1980 she became the administrator of the Pilates Studio. She taught faculty and students at SUNY at Purchase until 1988. She began teaching master classes in 1987 and started teaching at Dr. Sichels Chiropractic two years later. In 1994 Phoebe started a teacher- training program for Power Pilates with Susan Moran. Phoebe also teaches advanced students at the School of American Ballet.

Ellen Pilchik Kaldor, PT, CPS

Ellen has been a practicing physiotherapist for the past 14 years. She received her Masters in Physiotherapy from Emory University in Atlanta, Georgia, and has worked in many different settings in Israel, New York City and London. She is certified in cranial sacral therapy and is very interested in how the mind and body work together.

About the author

Caron Bosler received her Masters in Dance Studies from The Laban Centre, London. She started teaching Pilates at 17 years old during her undergraduate in Dance at SUNY at Purchase in New York. She has been certified in Pilates from the Pilates Studio in New York and Alan Herdman in London, as well as training under Romana Kryzanowska, Ron Flecher, and Raol Isacowitz. She has taught Pilates in numerous studios and gyms including: the Pilates Studio, Tribecca Bodyworks, Dr. Sichels Chiropractic, New York Sports Club, Alan Herdman Studios, the Laban Centre and Cristiane Dominici Studios. She has lectured and guest-taught in America, England and France.
Caron currently teaches privately in London and can be reached at: caronbosler@pilatesinternational.com

Acknowledgements

I would like to thank Sarah and David for giving me the opportunity to write this book. I would also like to thank the many teachers who have created lasting impressions on my beliefs and work. Thank you to Phoebe Higgins and Ellen Kaldor for all your dedication and scrutiny. Thank you to Alan Herdman, for expanding my mind and giving me so many opportunities. Thank you Elle for all the support across the miles. Thank you to Bustchops for doing just that whenever I take life too seriously. I love and appreciate you all!

Picture Credits

Picture p8 © I. C. Rapoport , Picture top p10 © Norman Eder , Picture bottom p11 © Getty images